T0227370

Advances in Coronary Angiography

Guest Editors

S. JAMES CHEN, PhD

JOHN D. CARROLL, MD

CARDIOLOGY CLINICS

www.cardiology.theclinics.com

Consulting Editor

MICHAEL H. CRAWFORD, MD

August 2009 • Volume 27 • Number 3

SAUNDERS an imprint of ELSEVIER, Inc.

W.B. SAUNDERS COMPANY
A Division of Elsevier Inc.

Elsevier, Inc. ● 1600 John F. Kennedy Blvd. ● Suite 1800 ● Philadelphia, Pennsylvania 19103-2899

http://www.theclinics.com

CARDIOLOGY CLINICS Volume 27, Number 3
August 2009 ISSN 0733-8651, ISBN-13: 978-1-4377-1197-4, ISBN-10: 1-4377-1197-9

Editor: Barbara Cohen-Kligerman

Cardiology Clinics (ISSN 0733-8651) is published quarterly by Elsevier Inc., 360 Park Avenue South, New York, NY 10010-1710. Months of issue are February, May, August, and November. Business and editorial Offices: 1600 John F. Kennedy Blvd., Suite 1800, Philadelphia, PA 19103-2899. Customer Service Office: 11830 Westline Industrial Drive, St. Louis, MO 63146. Periodicals postage paid at New York, NY, and additional mailing offices. Subscription prices are $244.00 per year for US individuals, $378.00 per year for US institutions, $122.00 per year for US students and residents, $298.00 per year for Canadian individuals, $470.00 per year for Canadian institutions, $346.00 per year for international individuals, $470.00 per year for international institutions and $173.00 per year for Canadian and foreign students/residents. To receive student/resident rate, orders must be accompanied by name of affiliated institution, data of term, and the signature of program/residency coordinator on institution letterhead. Orders will be billed at individual rate until proof of status is received. Foreign air speed delivery is included in all Clinics subscription prices. All prices are subject to change without notice. **POSTMASTER:** Send address changes to Cardiology Clinics, Elsevier Periodicals Customer Service, 11830 Westline Industrial Drive, St. Louis, MO 63146. **Customer Service: 1-800-654-2452 (US). From outside of the US, call 314-453-7041. Fax: 314-453-5170. E-mail: JournalsCustomer Service-usa@elsevier.com (for print support); JournalsOnlineSupport-usa@elsevier.com (for online support).**

Reprints. For copies of 100 or more, of articles in this publication, please contact the Commercial Reprints Department, Elsevier Inc., 360 Park Avenue South, New York, NY 10010-1710. Tel.: 212-633-3812; Fax: 212-462-1935; Email: reprints@elsevier.com.

Cardiology Clinics is also published in Spanish by McGraw-Hill Interamericana Editores S. A., P.O. Box 5-237, 06500, Mexico D. F., Mexico; in Portuguese by Reichmann and Alfonso Editores Rio de Janeiro, Brazil; and in Greek by Dimitrios P. Lagos, 8 Pondon Street, GR115-28 Ilissia, Greece.

Cardiology Clinics is covered in *MEDLINE/PubMed (Index Medicus), Excerpta Medica, The Cumulative Index to Nursing and Allied Health Literature* (CINAHL).

Printed and bound by CPI Group (UK) Ltd, Croydon, CR0 4YY

Transferred to Digital Print 2011

Contributors

CONSULTING EDITOR

MICHAEL H. CRAWFORD, MD
Professor of Medicine, University of California, San Francisco; Lucie Stern Chair in Cardiology, and Interim Chief of Cardiology, University of California, San Francisco Medical Center, San Francisco, California

GUEST EDITORS

S. JAMES CHEN, PhD
Associate Professor, Department of Medicine, Division of Cardiology, University of Colorado Denver, Aurora, Colorado

JOHN D. CARROLL, MD
Professor, Department of Medicine, Division of Cardiology, University of Colorado Denver, Aurora, Colorado

AUTHORS

NICO BRUINING, PhD
Department of Cardiology, Thorax Center, Erasmus Medical Center, Rotterdam, The Netherlands

EUGENIA P. CARROLL, MD
Assistant Professor, Department of Medicine, Division of Cardiology, University of Colorado Denver, Aurora, Colorado

JOHN D. CARROLL, MD
Professor, Department of Medicine, Division of Cardiology, University of Colorado Denver, Aurora, Colorado

IVAN P. CASSERLY, MB, BCh
Assistant Professor of Medicine, Division of Cardiology, Section of Interventional Cardiology, University of Colorado Denver School of Medicine, Aurora, Colorado

S. JAMES CHEN, PhD
Associate Professor, Department of Medicine, Division of Cardiology, University of Colorado Denver, Aurora, Colorado

SEBASTIAAN DE WINTER, BSc
Department of Cardiology, Thorax Center, Erasmus Medical Center, Rotterdam, The Netherlands

EFSTATHIOS P. EFSTATHOPOULOS, PhD
2nd Department of Radiology, Medical School, University of Athens, Athens, Greece

RAOUL FLORENT, MSc
Medisys Research Lab, Philips Healthcare, Suresnes, France

JOEL A. GARCIA, MD
Director, Catheterization Laboratory and Interventional Services, Division of Cardiology and Assistant Professor, Division of Cardiovascular Diseases and Interventional Cardiology, Denver Health Medical Center, University of Colorado Hospital at Denver and Health Sciences Center, Denver, Colorado

MICHAEL GRASS, PhD
Philips Technologie GmbH, Forschungslaboratorien, Germany

JOHN C. GURLEY, MD
Professor of Medicine, Division of
Cardiovascular Medicine, The Linda and Jack
Gill Heart Institute, University of Kentucky
Medical Center, Lexington, Kentucky

ADAM R. HANSGEN, BS
Senior Research Assistant, Department of
Medicine, Division of Cardiology, University
of Colorado Denver, Aurora, Colorado

HARVEY S. HECHT, MD
Chief, Cardiovascular Computed Tomography,
Department of Interventional Cardiology,
Lenox Hill Hospital, New York, New York

**DEMOSTHENES G. KATRITSIS, MD, PhD,
FRCP**
Department of Cardiology, Coronary Flow
Research Unit, Athens Euroclinic, Greece

ANDREW J.P. KLEIN, MD
Interventional Cardiology Staff, Division of
Cardiology, John Cochran Veterans Affairs
Medical Center; Assistant Professor of
Medicine, St. Louis University, St. Louis,
Missouri.

JOHN C. MESSENGER, MD
Associate Professor of Medicine, Division of
Cardiology, Section of Interventional
Cardiology, University of Colorado Denver
School of Medicine, Aurora, Colorado

**ANDREW D. MICHAELS, MD, MAS, FACC,
FAHA**
Associate Professor of Medicine and Director,
Division of Cardiology, Cardiac Catheterization
Laboratory and Interventional Cardiology,
University of Utah Health Sciences Center, Salt
Lake City, Utah

BABAK MOVASSAGHI, PhD
Clinical Scientist, Philips Cardiovascular X-ray,
Philips Healthcare, Denver, Colorado

ANNE NEUBAUER, PhD
Philips Research North America, Briarcliff
Manor, New York

IOANNIS PANTOS, MSc
Department of Cardiology, Coronary Flow
Research Unit, Athens Euroclinic; 2nd
Department of Radiology, Medical School,
University of Athens, Athens, Greece

R. KEVIN ROGERS, MD
Cardiology Fellow, Division of Cardiology,
University of Utah Health Sciences Center, Salt
Lake City, Utah

DANIEL RUIJTERS, MSc
Senior Scientist, Philips Healthcare, Cardio/
Vascular Innovation, Best, The Netherlands

DIRK SCHÄFER, PhD
Philips Research Europe, Tomographic
Imaging Systems, Hamburg, Germany

GERT SCHOONENBERG, MSc
Department of Cardiovascular Innovation,
Business Unit Cardio/Vascular X-Ray,
Philips Healthcare; Division Biomedical
Imaging and Modeling, Department
of Biomedical Engineering, Eindhoven
University of Technology, Eindhoven,
The Netherlands

PATRICK W. SERRUYS, MD, PhD
Department of Cardiology, Thorax Center,
Erasmus Medical Center, Rotterdam, The
Netherlands

ONNO WINK, PhD
Researcher Scientist, Philips Healthcare,
Cardio/Vascular X-ray, Aurora, Colorado

Contents

> Traditional coronary angiography presents a variety of limitations related to image acquisition, content, interpretation, and patient safety. These limitations were first apparent with coronary angiography used as a diagnostic tool and have been further magnified in today's world of percutaneous coronary intervention (PCI), with the frequent use of implantable coronary stents. Improvements are needed to overcome the limitations in using current two-dimensional radiographic imaging for optimizing patient selection, quantifying vessel features, guiding PCI, and assessing PCI results. Barriers to such improvements include the paucity of clinical outcomes studies related to new imaging technology, the resistance to changing long-standing practices, the need for physician and staff member training, and the costs associated with acquiring and effectively using these advances in coronary angiography.

Acquiring Images in Coronary Angiography

> Flat detectors are the heart of high-performance imaging systems that provide new capabilities as well as new hazards. The superior image quality enables operators to work with heavier patients and steeper projections. Under these conditions, exposure control computers automatically increase the production of x-rays to compensate for absorption by body tissues. Image quality is preserved, and operators may not be aware of the very high skin doses delivered during prolonged procedures. Although it is assumed that flat detector systems are safe, the potential for radiation overexposure and skin injury is real. This article examines the unique radiation hazards of flat detector fluoroscopy and suggests practical steps that clinicians can take to protect themselves and their patients from radiation injury.

> The numerous well-documented limitations of standard fixed-acquisition coronary angiography led to the development of rotational angiography. This acquisition method uses automated gantry movements while numerous angiographic projections are obtained, and thus overcomes many of the limitations of standard angiography. This article highlights the techniques, advantages, and disadvantages of each type of rotational angiography currently commercially available. Also included is a discussion of the evolution of rotational angiography, from its initial conception and pilot studies to its latest step forward on the developmental road towards enhanced coronary imaging.

enhancing techniques that provide improved stent visualization by eliminating motion artifact. These techniques can be useful in the detection of inadequate stent expansion. These motion-corrected x-ray stent (MXS) visualization techniques are more time-efficient compared to intravascular ultrasound (IVUS), require less training of catheterization laboratory personnel, and have lower procedural costs. However, little clinical or outcome data evidence exist for MXS. Though IVUS remains the gold standard for evaluation of the adequacy of stent expansion, MXS may be a viable adjunctive imaging tool in certain clinical scenarios.

Cardiology Clinics

VISIT THE CLINICS ONLINE!
Access your subscription at:
www.theclinics.com

Foreword

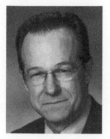

Michael H. Crawford, MD
Consulting Editor

While most cardiologists are excited about new 64- to 320-slice computed tomography images of the coronary arteries and the promise of magnetic resonance imaging for coronary visualization, the invasive cardiac catheterization laboratory has been evolving as well. Nothing stands still in medicine, and many important clinical issues are moving targets when it comes to research trials. Thus, I was delighted when Drs. Chen and Carroll agreed to guest edit this issue of *Cardiology Clinics* on the topic of Advances in Coronary Angiography. They have assembled an international group of experts on this topic. The excellent articles discuss image acquisition, digital processing, and the multimodality imaging aspects of coronary angiography. The latter is the new hot topic, but the economic issues surrounding multimodality imaging have not been fully worked out. Only recently did Medicare and some insurance companies start paying for coronary CT angiography in certain circumstances. For most symptomatic patients,

invasive coronary angiography remains the diagnostic technique of choice. In the future though, multimodality imaging performed in one laboratory makes sense and the issues surrounding this concept are discussed in the last section of this issue.

Everyone who performs or orders coronary angiography will enjoy this issue, which brings us up to date on the advances in cardiac catheterization–based coronary artery imaging and its relationship to newer, less invasive techniques.

Michael H. Crawford, MD
Division of Cardiology
Department of Medicine
University of California
San Francisco Medical Center
505 Parnassus Avenue, Box 0124
San Francisco, CA 94143-0124, USA

E-mail address:
crawfordm@medicine.ucsf.edu (M.H. Crawford)

Cardiol Clin 27 (2009) xi
doi:10.1016/j.ccl.2009.06.001
0733-8651/09/$ – see front matter © 2009 Elsevier Inc. All rights reserved.

cardiology.theclinics.com

Preface

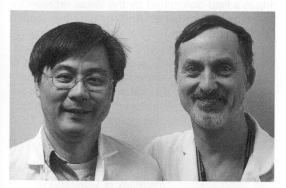

S. James Chen, PhD, John D. Carroll, MD
Guest Editors

This issue of *Cardiology Clinics* brings together contributions from around the world, investigators who are clinical versus imaging science in their orientation, and representatives from academic medical centers and the imaging industry. Each article is written to be accessible to those with a basic knowledge of coronary Imaging but also to be stimulating and educational to those who are experts and investigators in medical imaging.

Attention has been paid to acknowledging contributions and relevant products from medical imaging companies. Advances in coronary angiography can make an impact on patient care only if they are made available in medical imaging equipment and other products found in the cardiac catheterization laboratory. Potential biases of the authors are dealt with by acknowledging affiliations and industry support, by describing all products that are available, and by avoiding product names unless necessary for clarity and potential need of the readership.

This monograph is organized into three major sections. The first section has to do with the acquisition of coronary angiographic images. The first article provides a background regarding the known limitations of current techniques and technology and the barriers to implementing improvements. Dr. Gurley presents the recent advances in flat detector technology with the critically important related issue of radiation safety. The new method of acquisition, rotational angiography, is presented by Drs. Klein and Garcia, two investigators with extensive practical knowledge. Drs. Messenger and Casserly of the University of

Colorado describe the techniques and products associated with catheter-based angiography, including the use of catheters, contrast media, and injection systems.

The second section covers where advances have been dramatic in the past decade and shows the major contributions of the imaging scientists and engineers from both academia and industry. Drs. Chen and Schäfer describe the modeling approach to produce a three-dimensional (3-D) representation of a patient's coronary tree from x-ray projection images. Subsequently, the multi-national investigative team of Schoonenberg, Neubauer, and Grass show us the future with 3-D reconstruction techniques that will soon make the transition from imaging laboratory to clinical practice. Visualization of coronary arteries in 3-D is an exciting development in coronary angiography that has now led to enhanced visualization of what is done to treat the patient, including implantation of cardiovascular devices. The academic clinical team from the University of Utah, Drs. Rogers and Michaels, review their work and that of others on clinical aspects of enhanced coronary stent visualization. Subsequently, Schoonenberg and Florent show us the future in 3-D stent and other device visualization using rotational acquisitions.

The third section has an emphasis on quantification, multimodality integration, and other futuristic aspects of coronary angiography. Drs. Pantos, Efstathopoulos, and Katritsis from Athens describe the approach to both traditional 2-D quantitative coronary angiography (QCA) and 3-D

Cardiol Clin 27 (2009) xiii–xiv
doi:10.1016/j.ccl.2009.04.006
0733-8651/09/$ – see front matter © 2009 Elsevier Inc. All rights reserved.

QCA. Then Drs. Garcia and Movassaghi, a clinical investigator and an imaging scientist, present how computer applications can help the physician solve the imaging tasks inherent in the performance and interpretation of coronary angiography data. The next article deals with the need, the technology, and the initial experience in integrating computer tomographic angiography (CTA) into the work flow and performance of percutaneous coronary intervention (PCI). The multidisciplinary team of Drs. Wink, Hecht, and Ruijters provide the expertise of imaging scientists and a clinical CTA leader. Similarly, the Rotterdam group (Drs. Bruining, de Winter, and Serruys) present their work and that of others in the integration of intravascular ultrasound (IVUS) into the angiographic suite with true fusion of both kinds of images. Dr. James Chen, Adam Hansgen, and Dr. John Carroll close with a look into emerging technologies and applications that will define the cardiac catheterization laboratory of the not-too-distant future.

Advances in coronary angiography are occurring in a field dominated by the visual representation of moving objects. Angiography has moved from the black-and-white projection image to complementary color-coded computer graphics. We, as editors, greatly appreciate the support of Elsevier in allowing the authors to illustrate with color images and to include movies that can be accessed in the online version of this issue at http://www.cardiology.theclinics.com.

S. James Chen, PhD

John D. Carroll, MD
University of Colorado Denver
Cardiac and Vascular Center
Leprino Building, 5th Floor, #519
12401 E. 17th Avenue, B-132
Aurora, CO 80045

E-mail addresses:
James.Chen@ucdenver.edu (S.J. Chen)
John.Carroll@ucdenver.edu (J.D. Carroll)

Coronary Angiography: The Need for Improvement and the Barriers to Adoption of New Technology

John D. Carroll, MD*, Eugenia P. Carroll, MD, S. James Chen, PhD

KEYWORDS
- Coronary angiography
- Percutaneous coronary intervention
- Coronary artery disease • Fluoroscopy • Stent • Radiation

Catheter-based coronary angiography has been a clinical tool for more than five decades.[1,2] Despite the development of other imaging techniques, including CT and MRI, selective (ie, catheter-based) radiographic coronary angiography still remains the most commonly performed method for imaging of the entire coronary tree.[3–5] The technology is widely available, there are many cardiologists well trained in the technique and the image interpretation, the spatial and temporal resolution are unsurpassed, and the diagnostic procedure can be easily transitioned into a therapeutic procedure. In addition to providing specific anatomic information, angiography also has an important prognostic role in the identification of coronary artery disease and the associated risk of subsequent morbidity and mortality.[6–9] The number of diagnostic and therapeutic angiographic procedures has increased dramatically during the last several decades. Catheter-based coronary angiography, with its two-dimensional (2D) projection images, will continue to be widely used, but the limitations must be recognized and improvements must be sought. New approaches involving image processing, quantitative analysis, and other imaging modalities combined with radiography are essential to advance the field and improve patient care. **Table 1** summarizes these limitations and directs the reader to articles in this issue that address these limitations through the use of new techniques and technology.

LIMITATIONS OF CURRENT APPROACHES AND TECHNOLOGY

A major goal of anatomically based medical imaging modalities is to accurately represent the imaging target. The 2D projection image of the coronary artery tree clearly falls short of the goal of representing the three-dimensional (3D) coronary tree. Over decades of use and experience, the cardiovascular community has lived with this limitation, but it must be explicitly recognized that this central limitation no longer has to be accepted because 3D technology is now available for radiographic coronary imaging, and it has become standard in CT and MRI imaging of the coronary tree.

The transition from 2D to 3D imaging must occur with attention to work flow and workloads. As outlined in **Table 1**, coronary angiography that produces 2D projection images has limitations related to how it is acquired, the nature of projection images, and the need for the operator to solve all the imaging tasks, such as obtaining views without vessel overlap and foreshortening in all vessel segments. The operator's workload has

Division of Cardiology, Department of Medicine, University of Colorado Denver, Leprino Office Building, Mail Stop B132, 12401 East 17th Avenue, Aurora, CO 80045, USA
* Corresponding author.
E-mail address: john.carroll@ucdenver.edu (J.D. Carroll).

Cardiol Clin 27 (2009) 373–383
doi:10.1016/j.ccl.2009.03.001

Table 1
Major clinical limitations of catheter-based coronary angiography

Category	Limitations	Articles Addressing Limitations
1. Safety: invasiveness	Requires vascular access and navigation back to coronary take-offs.	Article 5
2. Safety: ionizing radiation	Substantial radiation given with diagnostic and interventional use.	Articles 2, 3, 6, 7, 11
3. Safety: contrast media	Use of angiographic dye with potential nephrotoxicty, especially for patients who have preexistent renal impairment.	Articles 2, 3, 4, 6, 7, 11
4. Technique of acquisition	Lack of standardization to achieve complete diagnostic study or focused PCI imaging. Operator-dependent selection of variable number of fixed projection views to avoid vessel overlap and minimize lesion foreshortening.	Articles 3, 11, 12
5. Image format	2D projection images, with inherent problems of foreshortening, overlap, and misrepresentation of key anatomic features such as lesion length, bifurcation angles, and tortuosity.	Articles 2, 3, 6, 7, 9, 10, 11, 12
6. Angiographic visualization	Visualization of lumen provides minimal information on vessel wall, which can lead to underestimation of disease. Limitations of hand injection of contrast.	Articles 2, 3, 4, 12, 13
7. Interpretation and analysis	Subjective and semiquantitative analysis using only those views acquired.	Articles 2, 6, 7, 8, 9, 10, 11
8. Advanced applications	2D format makes images unsuitable for fusion with IVUS or other datasets and prevents use in advanced guidance systems	Articles 9, 10, 11, 12, 13

increased from the days of diagnostic coronary angiography to today's use today of percutaneous coronary intervention (PCI), which often involves the simultaneous care of critically ill patients. In planning innovations and advances in coronary angiography, a major design and performance parameter is the reduction of operator workload through automation, computer guidance, and providing tools that are simple to use.

Traditional angiography is fundamentally limited by its 2D representation of 3D structures and the consequent imaging artifacts that impair optimal visualization. Misrepresentations of 3D coronary features include such important measurements as lesion length, angles of bifurcations, and vessel curvature, or tortuosity. It should be noted that all these geometric features are included in lesion classification systems used to describe anatomy and predict success versus failure and complications in PCI.

Specifically, the use of 2D projection images may lead to important clinical mistakes in assessing lesion length (**Fig. 1**). The source of error is generally related to two factors: the degree of foreshortening of the lesion in the projection image and the scaling factor used. Vessel foreshortening is often unappreciated, and even experienced interventional cardiologists often choose a working view that has substantial foreshortening.[10] Scaling factor errors arise when the calibration object, typically the distal end of a catheter, lies in a different plane than the lesion relative to the distance from the radiation source. In **Table 2**, examples are given of how these two errors can result in significant underestimation of the true length of a 15-mm lesion. The degree of error is greater with longer lesions and when lesions traverse curvilinear vascular segments. Interventionalists try to overcome this limitation by using the distance between markers on a balloon angioplasty catheter that is placed across the lesion to estimate lesion length and to select the proper stent length.

Standard 2D projection images also misrepresent bifurcation and take-off angles. Measuring angles in an image can lead to either over- or underestimating the true angle (**Fig. 2**). The angle of origin of a branch has a variety of clinical ramifications for endovascular interventions. For example, the ability to access a side branch using a guide wire or to advance a delivery system is partially determined by the take-off angle. An understanding of the branching angle is important in assessing the likelihood of plaque shifting into a vessel as the result of placing stents up to the ostium of a branch. The emerging use of bifurcation stents will increase the need to better understand and quantify branching anatomy in terms of the risk of failure and the procedural difficulty, the choice of device size and configuration, and the alteration of the bifurcation anatomy by using the implanted device. Presently, bifurcation stenting technique has been built on the limitations of single stents and the use of 2D images. The simplistic system classifies bifurcations as being Y-shaped if the angle between the branches is less than 70° and as being T-shaped if the angulation is less than 70°.[11]

The degree of vessel curvature is another clinically relevant anatomic feature of the coronary tree (**Box 1**). Unfortunately, curvature is often misrepresented and poorly quantified using 2D projection images, for several reasons. First, the perceived degree of vessel curvature is projection-view dependent (**Fig. 3**). Second, the means of quantifying vessel curvature are primitive if done using projection images. It is striking that in many stent studies, tortuosity is quantified on a scale of being slight, medium, and marked because no quantitative tools have been available. Third and finally, coronary shape is not static but varies throughout the cardiac cycle.[12] The coronary arteries are affixed to the underlying myocardium. Any method that attempts to analyze coronary arterial shape deformations should include descriptions that account for the dynamic shape change during the cardiac cycle. The 3D models of coronary arterial trees created from coronary angiographic data represent the true coronary anatomy and allow quantification of tortuosity for clinical purpose and study shape changes caused by stent-vessel interactions.[13]

The lack of calibration in most clinically acquired coronary images further confounds the limitations of using 2D projection images to accurately quantify these key anatomic features. Despite the ability of most modern angiographic systems to provide automated and internal calibration of images (ie, true distance per pixel), this is rarely done because it necessitates first placing the patient's heart in isocenter by moving the table height and horizontal positioning. By not placing the heart in isocenter, the operator must otherwise spend additional time manually designating a calibration object to use in performing quantitative coronary analysis (QCA) of vessel diameters and lesion lengths.

It is useful to reconsider the limitations of traditional coronary angiography from the perspective of interventional cardiology and the need to safely, effectively, and efficiently place stents to treat lesions. First, we must recognize the limitation that coronary angiography is "lumenology" and that the incorporation of intra-vascular ultrasound (IVUS) and computed tomography angiography (CTA) into the coronary study may be important. Additional limitations of traditional coronary angiography relate to the optimization of stent selection, delivery, and placement. Traditional 2D projection images often provide an underestimation of the length of a stent that is needed to cover a lesion because of unappreciated foreshortening. In **Table 3**, the many clinical needs for imaging related to the use of coronary stents are described. The table also provides a comparison of current approaches and new imaging technologies to address the current clinical problems in coronary stent implantation. Finally, the table refers readers to other articles in this issue that describe these concerns and new techniques and technologies that may meet these clinical needs.

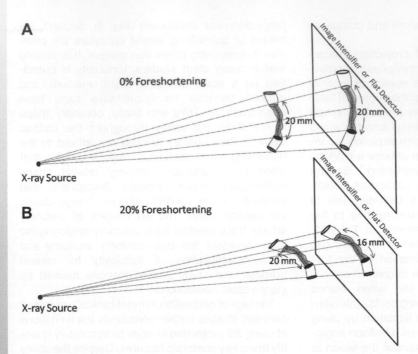

A

0% Foreshortening

20 mm

20 mm

X-ray Source

Image Intensifier or Flat Detector

B

20% Foreshortening

16 mm

20 mm

X-ray Source

Image Intensifier or Flat Detector

Fig. 1. Simplified model of foreshortening. (*A*) Perpendicular orientation of the radiographic beam to a vessel segment or lesion of interest results in minimal distortion of the projection image. (*B*) Without perpendicular radiography beam alignment, vessel foreshortening occurs and results in suboptimal projection images that misrepresent the true length of a lesion or vessel segment.

Also, the use of 2D projection images severely limits the introduction of new technologies such as image fusion and robotic guidance systems. The registration of an intravascular ultrasound acquisition on a 2D projection image is much more difficult than on a 3D representation of the coronary data. Likewise, guidance systems must be driven by a 3D representation of the anatomic system. Therefore, the transition to 3D angiographic data is a first step and is critical to enabling other developments in imaging and image guidance of interventions.

In summary, the multiple limitations of traditional coronary angiography are clear. It is also evident that multiple "work-arounds" have been devised by angiographers over the decades. These solutions are far from perfect because they require the operator to assume a large workload and a high level of expertise in using imperfect representations of coronary arteries.

The major burden of the limitations of 2D images falls on the patient. Radiation exposure and contrast volumes are high when the angiographer must search for a "good view." The patient's burden is even higher when a PCI is prolonged because of poor visualization of key anatomic features, mistakes in understanding complex anatomy, and placement of stents using suboptimal working views that misrepresent the location of an ostium and other features.

BARRIERS TO THE ADOPTION OF NEW TECHNIQUES AND TECHNOLOGIES

The advances in coronary angiography presented in the other articles in this issue involve changes in how images are acquired, processed, displayed, and used by the clinician. When, how widely, and how rapidly will these new

Table 2
Mistakes in lesion-length assessment in 2D images

True Lesion Length (mm)	Foreshortening Error (%)	Scaling Factor Error (%)	Assessed Lesion Length in 2D Projection Image (mm)
15	0	0	15
15	33	0	10
15	0	20	12.75
15	33	20	9

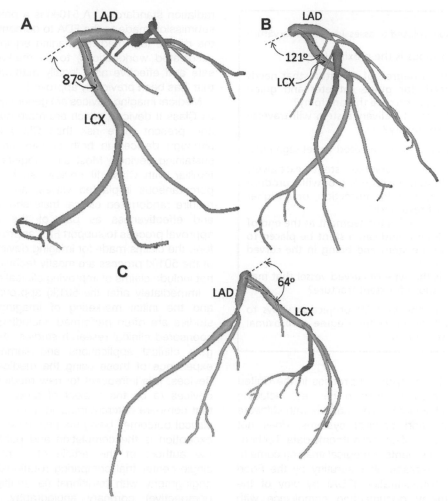

Fig. 2. Angiographic view dependency of bifurcation angle measurement. View of the LCX bifurcation angle (true 3D bifurcation angle = 87°) resulting from (A) the correctly estimated bifurcation angle, (B) the overestimated bifurcation angle, and (C) the underestimated bifurcation angle. LAD, left anterior descending artery; LCX, left circumflex artery.

technologies be incorporated into the thousands of cardiac catheterization laboratories around the world? Will some of the technologies be adopted at all? In **Table 4**, the major barriers to change in the cardiac catheterization room and some potential solutions to overcoming these barriers are outlined. These barriers must be overcome to acquire and effectively use these new techniques and technologies. Indeed, it is not uncommon to already see new angiographic systems installed with many advanced features that are rarely, if ever, used.

The first and most compelling resistance to changing the techniques and technology in coronary angiography is the need to answer the two fundamental questions of why should there be any change and whether a change is clearly an

advancement. As previously discussed in this article, there are multiple limitations of traditional 2D projection images. Most importantly and immediately, there are compelling reasons to seek new techniques and tools that will reduce the radiation dose and the contrast volume to the patient. In addition, there are numerous examples in which mistakes and uncertainties in PCI performance could be addressed by using more advanced technology.

If there is agreement that the current techniques and technologies in coronary angiography have limitations and are problematic in certain aspects of patient care, then the next step is to prove that the new proposed techniques and technologies are better and provide true advancements in patient care.

Box 1
Clinical issues related to assessing vessel curvature

1. How tortuous is the proximal vessel?

    a. Is this a degree of curvature that needs a particular guide catheter and guide wire to overcome this anatomy?
    b. What stent delivery system will traverse this tortuosity?

2. How curved is the diseased vessel segment?

    a. Will an implanted stent excessively straighten the segment, or will it produce a kink, an edge dissection, or a higher rate of restenosis?
    b. How curved is the segment at the end of the lesion, and can a stent be placed to avoid the stent end being in the curved segment?
    c. Is this the type of curved vessel that may predispose for stent fracture?

3. What are the best 2D projection views to optimally visualize the degree of proximal and distal curvature?

The regulatory approval process in the United States for medical imaging devices, including radiographic systems, workstations with software applications, and archival systems, does not provide this type of clinical outcome data. Technological advancements in medical imaging come to the US marketplace after scrutiny by the Food and Drug Administration (FDA) by way of the 501(k) pathway documenting compliance with general technical performance measures, good manufacturing practice, labeling, prohibitions against misbranding and adulteration, and

radiation standards.[14] A 510(k) is a premarketing submission made to the FDA to demonstrate that the device (eg, medical imaging equipment and associated workstations) to be marketed is as safe and effective as a legally marketed device that has been previously approved.

Medical imaging devices are generally classified as Class II devices, which are more complicated and present more risk than Class I devices, although devices in both classes are not life-sustaining devices. Most cardiologists are more familiar with Class III devices such as stents, percutaneous implanted valves, and such that require randomized clinical trials showing safety and effectiveness as part of the premarket approval process to support FDA approval. Therefore, the claims made for imaging devices as part of the 501(k) process are mostly technical and do not include claims of improving clinical outcomes.

Immediately after the 501(k) approval process and the initial marketing of imaging devices, studies are often performed, including industry-sponsored clinical research studies, that investigate clinical applications and summarize the experience of those using the medical imaging devices. It is infrequent for new medical imaging devices to be the subject of randomized trials that compare different imaging devices and have clinical outcomes being the primary endpoint. An exception is the completion and publication by the authors of this article of a randomized, single-center trial comparing rotational coronary angiography with traditional (ie, multiple, fixed-perspective) coronary angiography. The trial demonstrated a substantial reduction in radiation exposure and contrast volume for patients.[15] It is often difficult, especially with the limited funding

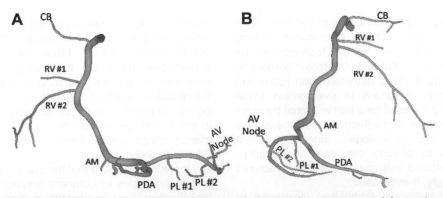

Fig. 3. View of angle dependency of the degree of vessel curvature. Right coronary arterial tree visualized at two different angiographic views in which the arterial segment of the main right coronary artery between the RV #2 and the PDA in (*A*) shows less tortuous shape than the same arterial segment in (*B*). AM, acute marginal branch; AV Node, atrioventricular node; CB, conus branch; PDA, posterior descending artery; PL, posterior lateral branch; RV, right ventricular branch.

available, to perform large, multicenter studies. Furthermore, it is challenging to design studies that isolate the impact of a new variation of an imaging device related to the clinical outcomes of a percutaneous intervention because so many other factors go into determining outcome. Therefore, studies often look at validation compared with alternative technologies, such as comparing radiographic stent visualization enhancement to intravascular ultrasound assessment of stent expansion.[16] Studies have also reported on the intermediate endpoints that may lead to improved clinical outcomes, such as the image content of rotational coronary angiographic images compared with images from a multiple, fixed-view perspective technique.[17]

As a result of the paucity of clinical studies of imaging-related impact on clinical outcomes, physicians and hospital administrators must evaluate new medical imaging systems and rely on their own assessment of potential clinical value and enhanced efficiency. Site visits to institutions that have used the technology also play a role in this assessment. Therefore, a barrier to advances in coronary angiography being adopted is the paucity and delayed nature of clinical outcome studies. This, coupled with the slow, cyclical, and often laborious capital purchasing process in hospitals, results in a slow rate of penetration of new imaging technologies as compared with that of therapeutic medical devices.

Even after acknowledging the need for change and demonstrating the proven benefit, there are additional barriers to overcome. A key one is individual and institutional resistance to change. The natural human reaction is to resist change, and there is no reason to believe that there is not resistance to change in health care in general and in the cardiac catheterization laboratory specifically.

Resistance to change, especially when it requires new skills and a change in work flow, uses a variety of rationales. Some will always feel that traditional coronary angiography meets their needs and will not acknowledge its limitations and their unmet needs. Others will resist change because they feel overwhelmed by the increasing complexity of medicine and the burden of keeping up with new knowledge. Some will invoke the time, pain, and expense needed to acquire new skills to effectively use new technologies. Indeed, some of the techniques and technologies presented in this issue require a substantial training phase and major capital purchases. Prior advances in imaging for the cardiac catheterization laboratory such as digital archiving and flat detectors did not have this barrier to change and were adopted without the need for new skills and changes in work flow.

The training needed as part of adopting the advances in coronary angiography described in this article ranges from being simple and straightforward to learning a fundamentally different approach for performing diagnostic coronary angiography and using radiographic technology to plan and execute PCI. For example, learning how to isocenter the patient's heart in the radiographic system is straightforward but has never been a task routinely performed in the past. Using processed radiographic images in the form of 3D models and reconstructions to plan and execute PCI is fundamentally different from the traditional method of using playback of acquired 2D cine-angiographic runs to plan PCI. Therefore, there is often a need to train physicians and other staff members in new techniques and technologies that involves more time and effort than the technology upgrades of the past. Cardiology training programs will be one avenue, but they are clearly inadequate for the large base of practicing cardiologists and the staff members in thousands of hospitals.

The effectiveness of training in these new techniques and technologies may require more than a vendor's trainer focusing on how to perform the technical steps (ie, the "buttonology"). Rather, clinical training is often needed to demonstrate the clinical value and show how the technology can be integrated into work flow and used in clinical care.

Streamlining of training can also be achieved if the technology has minimal user interaction. The adoption of coronary modeling applications requires training to perform the sequential steps required of the user to produce a model. Removing the user from this process by automation, as used with coronary reconstruction technology, may lead to a reduction in training burden and expense, and wider adoption and more frequent use of technology.

The final barriers to change are the cost of the technology and the cost of training to effectively use the new technology. New medical technology typically comes with an increased cost. The major cost has usually been for the radiographic system, but now peripherals such as workstations loaded with applications, automatic injectors, and large flat screens present additional costs. The process of capital purchasing in hospitals is subject to a variety of factors beyond the scope of this article. Major opportunities for hospitals, physicians, and staff members to improve coronary imaging are linked to the capital purchasing cycle. At the time this article was written, the world economy was in a recession, and the ability of health care systems to bring new technology to patients was likely to be slowed by this broad economic factor.

Table 3
Coronary angiographic needs related to PCI using coronary stents

Stent-related Considerations	Resultant Clinical Problems	Current Technology or Approaches	New Imaging Technology to Address Problems	Articles Related to Problems
Stent selection: diameter and length	Undersizing and oversizing may cause clinical events	"Eyeball" estimates of needed stent size and 2D QCA. Trial-and-error approach.	3D quantitative assessment of anatomy and use of CTA/IVUS insights	Articles 6, 7, 8, 9, 10, 11, 12, 13
Stent selection: degree of conformability	Stents may straighten arteries and cause edge lesions	General knowledge that kinks may occur when vessels are curved.	3D quantitative assessment of curvature and threshold detection when a more-conformable design is needed	Articles 3, 6, 7, 10, 11, 12
Stent delivery system performance	Failure to reach lesion	Try a system and see if it reaches the lesion.	Advanced 3D analysis of pathway to lesion plus assessment of vessel rigidity	Articles 6, 7, 10, 11, 12, 13
Placement of stent	Geographic miss	Use a 2D projection view that shows the entire lesion.	Optimal view for stent placement using computer analysis of 3D tree data	Articles 3, 6, 7, 8, 9, 10, 11, 12
Visualization of implanted stent	Thinner struts and larger patients lead to poor visibility	Use high-dose cine-acquisitions in multiple views.	Stent visualization enhancement technologies as in-room tools	Articles 2, 8, 9, 12

Assessment of expansion/wall apposition	Poor expansion and apposition lead to thrombosis and restenosis	Use noncompliant balloons and perform routine postdilatation or use IVUS.	Quantitative stent visualization enhancement fused with angiography directs need for further stent expansion	Articles 8 and 9
Long-term assessment of stent durability	Stent fracture is not rare and leads to restenosis and clinical events	Look for stent fracture with gross strut separation in patients who have restenosis.	Quantitative 3D stent visualization technologies using markers embedded on stents to detect most subtle forms of fracture	Articles 8 and 9
Development of new stent designs	Poor understanding of in vivo human device-vessel interactions blocks improvement	2D angiographic data, with all its limitations.	Quantitative assessment of stent-vessel interaction using 3D data and advanced analysis	Articles 6 and 7

Table 4
Barriers to adaptation of advances in coronary angiography

Barriers	Possible Solutions
Evidence-based medicine	• Perform and distribute postmarketing studies that address clinical validation and impact on patient care
Culture and work flow changes	• Identify local champions • Demonstrate the need for change • Involve staff members
Training of physicians and staff	• Engage cardiology departments in training programs • Offer continuing medical education programs • Provide hands-on industry training at clinical sites
Financial considerations	• Articulate clinical justification and business plan for capital purchase committees

The cost of training is clearly greater when new skills and knowledge must be acquired and the technology causes a fundamental change in the way procedures are performed. Such more-advanced and clinically based training is inherently more expensive, typically done off-site, and requires physicians and staff members to be away from their practices. If training is made an option in the capital purchase order, then it may be perceived as optional and expendable.

In conclusion, the barriers for adopting the new techniques and technologies described in this article are numerous. The barriers must be explicitly identified and overcome. The major motivating factors that will cause individuals and institutions to overcome these barriers are improving patient outcomes and reducing risks. The proof and supporting evidence that these major new technologies have a clinical value worth the cost typically is found after the product is approved and released. Scientifically gathered data from well-designed clinical investigation then provides the documentation of improved quality of patient care.

REFERENCES

1. Radner S. Attempt at roentgenologic visualization of coronary blood vessels in man. Acta Radiol 1945;26: 497–502.
2. Sones FM Jr, Shirey EK. Cine coronary arteriography. Mod Concepts Cardiovasc Dis 1962;31: 735–8.
3. Kim WY, Danias PG, Stuber M, et al. Coronary magnetic resonance angiography for the detection of coronary stenoses. N Engl J Med 2001;345: 1863–9.
4. Achenbach S, Giesler T, Ropers D, et al. Detection of coronary artery stenoses by contrast-enhanced, retrospectively electrocardiographically gated, multislice spiral computed tomography. Circulation 2001;103:2535–8.
5. Achenbach S, Moshage W, Ropers D, et al. Value of electronbeam computed tomography for the noninvasive detection of high-grade coronary artery stenoses and occlusions. N Engl J Med 1998;339: 1964–71.
6. Friesinger GC, Page EE, Ross RS. Prognostic significance of coronary arteriography. Trans Assoc Am Physicians 1970;83:78–92.
7. Oberman A, Jones WB, Riley CP, et al. Natural history of coronary artery disease. Bull N Y Acad Med 1972;48:1109–25.
8. Bruschke AV, Proudfit WL, Sones FM. Progress study of 590 consecutive non-surgical cases of coronary disease followed for 5 to 9 years. I: arterographic correlations. Circulation 1973;47:1147–53.
9. Scanlon PJ, Faxon DP, Audet AM, et al. ACC/AHA guidelines for coronary angiography: a report of the American College of Cardiology/American Heart Association Task Force on Practice Guidelines (Committee on Coronary Angiography). J Am Coll Cardiol 1999;33:1756–824.
10. Green NE, Chen SY, Hansgen AR, et al. Angiographic views used for percutaneous coronary interventions: a three-dimensional analysis of physician-determined vs. computer-generated views. Catheter Cardiovasc Interv 2005;64:451–9.
11. Iakovou I, Ge L, Colombo A. Contemporary stent treatment of coronary bifurcations. J Am Coll Cardiol 2005;46:1446–55.
12. Liao R, Messenger JC, Chen SY, et al. Four-dimensional analysis of cyclic changes in coronary artery shape. Catheter Cardiovasc Interv 2002;55(3): 344–54.
13. Liao R, Chen SY, Green NE, et al. Three-dimensional analysis of in vivo coronary stent–coronary vessel interactions. Int J Cardiovasc Imaging 2004;20:305–13.
14. U.S. Food and Drug Administration. Available at: http://www.fda.gov/cdrh/. Accessed April 30, 2009.

15. Maddux JT, Wink O, Messenger JC, et al. Randomized study of the safety and clinical utility of rotational angiography versus standard angiography in the diagnosis of coronary artery disease. Catheter Cardiovasc Interv 2004;62:167–74.

16. Mishell JM, Vakharia KT, Ports TA, et al. Determination of adequate coronary stent expansion using StentBoost, a novel fluoroscopic image processing technique. Catheter Cardiovasc Interv 2007;69:84–93.

17. Garcia J, Agostoni KT, Green NE, et al. Rotational vs. standard coronary angiography: an image content analysis. in press. Catheter Cardiovasc Interv 2009;73(6):753–61.

Flat Detectors and New Aspects of Radiation Safety

John C. Gurley, MD

KEYWORDS

- Flat detector • Fluoroscopy • Radiation safety
- Catheterization laboratory • X-ray dose monitoring

Flat detector (FD) fluoroscopy systems have largely replaced image intensifiers in the modern catheterization laboratory, and for good reason. Flat detectors produce stable, distortion-free images with extended dynamic range. These attributes are necessary for advanced image-processing techniques such as stent enhancement, 3-dimensional (3D) roadmapping, and soft tissue imaging. In addition, FD systems give clinicians a high-performance tool for standard interventional fluoroscopy. The superior contrast resolution and improved x-ray detection allow operators to work with heavier patients and steeper projections than were previously possible. But this enhanced capability is not without risk.

It is a myth that radiation injuries are caused by old or improperly calibrated x-ray equipment. Modern FD systems incorporate many refinements that can help minimize x-ray exposure, but the radiation output needed to produce a useful coronary image is not much different than it was with image intensifier systems of generations past. State-of-the-art FD systems are more than capable of causing serious injury (**Fig. 1**).

If anything, the risk of radiation injury in the flat detector era has paradoxically *increased*. This is in part a result of the expanding scope and complexity of interventional procedures, such as occluded-vessel intervention, that can require prolonged fluoroscopy. It is also a result of FD technology itself, which can enable operators to work under difficult imaging conditions that require high radiation doses. Finally, fluoroscopy has become so fundamental to procedural cardiology that some practitioners have developed a casual attitude toward radiation safety. Operators can wrongly assume that the government would not allow manufacturers to sell unsafe equipment, and that hospital physicists will be responsible for safety inspections and dose monitoring.

FLAT DETECTORS AND THE PARADOXIC DOSE HAZARD

Flat detectors excel at converting x-ray photons into useful images. This is mainly the result of their greater sensitivity to x-rays (higher quantum detection efficiency) and superior grayscale resolution. These advantages allow FD systems to provide usable images under conditions where x-ray penetration is most difficult—in heavy patients and in steep projections. But there may be a price to pay for this improved capacity.

The absorption of x-ray energy by body tissue is nonlinear, which means that heavy patients require disproportionately large entry doses to generate the image. For each additional centimeter of tissue penetrated, the input dose must be increased by about 25% (**Table 1**). Adding only 3 cm of tissue thickness can require twice the input dose, and 8 cm of tissue can require 6 times the dose. Steep angles of view increase the x-ray beam path and require similar dose increases (**Fig. 2**). Unfortunately, the operator may not always be aware of these situations that call for high dose rates.

A hazard arises when (1) a fluoroscopy system can *automatically* produce large amounts of radiation to overcome thick tissue paths; (2) a superior

The Linda and Jack Gill Heart Institute, University of Kentucky Medical Center, 760 South Limestone Street, Lexington, KY 40513, USA
E-mail address: jcgurl0@uky.edu

Cardiol Clin 27 (2009) 385–394
doi:10.1016/j.ccl.2009.04.004
0733-8651/09/$ – see front matter © 2009 Elsevier Inc. All rights reserved.

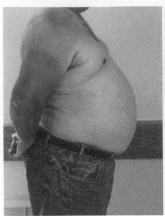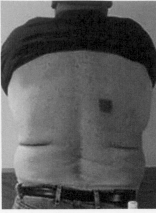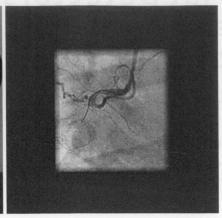

Fig. 1. Significant radiation skin injury following occluded-vessel intervention in a properly maintained FD catheterization laboratory. Factors contributing to the injury included obesity and prolonged procedure time.

detector can supply acceptable images under difficult conditions; and (3) the system fails to notify the operator when high dose rates are being delivered. All of these conditions exist in the typical FD catheterization laboratory.

A modern FD catheterization laboratory is highly automated. The operator simply steps on a pedal to display images of consistent brightness, regardless of patient size or projection. An exposure control computer manipulates peak kilovoltage (kVp), filament current (mA), and pulse width to produce an optimized image. When large patients or dense tissues are encountered, the system automatically produces more x-rays and more penetrating x-rays. If the resulting image is acceptable, operators can work for extended periods, while unwittingly delivering very large doses of radiation to the patient's skin.

EVIDENCE FOR THE DOSE HAZARD

We have examined the relationship between image quality and x-ray dose for matching FD and image intensifier–based catheterization laboratories. These catheterization laboratories were produced by the same manufacturer (Philips Medical Systems). They used the same x-ray tube, frame rate, fields of view, and nominal exposure settings. The only difference was the type of detector. Measurements of x-ray dose and image quality were obtained under identical imaging conditions, with simulated patients of varying size.

Image quality measurements were obtained with a NEMA XR21-2000 phantom that had been modified to simulate very heavy patients.[1,2] This phantom used 10-, 20-, 30-, 37.5-, and 42.5-cm thicknesses of acrylic, which has x-ray absorption and scatter properties similar to soft tissue. High-contrast spatial resolution was measured with

a line-pair (LP) phantom embedded in the acrylic block. Low-contrast resolution was assessed with iodine-filled chambers simulating contrast-filled vessels of varying size and opacity. The visibility of moving structures was assessed with a rotating disk containing wire spokes of different diameters. X-ray doses were measured with an ionization chamber.

The relationship between image quality and x-ray dose can be illustrated by the nomograms in **Figs. 3–6**. Image quality is plotted on the vertical axis and attenuator thickness on the horizontal axis. X-ray doses are plotted on the secondary vertical axis.

Contrast Resolution

For both FD and image intensifier (II) fluoroscopy, the ability to detect low-contrast objects fell linearly with increasing attenuator thickness, but the fall-off was more gradual with FD fluoroscopy.

Table 1
Relationship between tissue thickness and expected input dose

Increase in Tissue Thickness, cm	Expected Input Dose, %
+ 1	25
+ 2	56
+ 3	95
+ 4	244
+ 5	305
+ 6	381
+ 7	477
+ 8	596

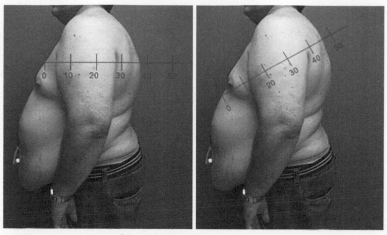

Fig. 2. Steep projections increase beam path and input dose. In this example, 30 degrees of caudal angle would increase the beam path by +7 cm, and would probably demand maximum output from the x-ray tube.

X-ray doses increased disproportionately as the system approached its maximum capacity. As shown in **Fig. 3**, the II system reached a 10-unit contrast threshold after penetrating 26.6 cm of acrylic with 5.4 R/minute entry dose. The FD system reached the same 10-unit contrast threshold at 33.7 cm (27% thicker), while delivering 12.1 R/minute (2.2 times greater dose).

Spatial Resolution

For II fluoroscopy, high-contrast spatial resolution dropped progressively from 3.4 to 2.5 LP/mm as attenuator thickness increased from 10 through 30 cm. For FD fluoroscopy, high-contrast spatial resolution was maintained at 3.1 LP/mm with attenuator thicknesses from 10 through 30 cm. Although both systems lost spatial resolution at

attenuator thicknesses greater than 30 cm, FD fluoroscopy performed better. As shown in **Fig. 4**, the II system resolved 2.5 LP/mm when penetrating 30 cm of acrylic, with a dose of 6.7 R/min. The FD system resolved 2.5 LP/mm when penetrating 37.5 cm of acrylic (25% thicker) with 15.5 R/minute (2.3 times greater dose). Again, FD fluoroscopy performed better with thick attenuators, but with escalating x-ray doses.

Motion Detection

As shown in **Fig. 5**, the II system reached an arbitrary threshold of 1.5 units after penetrating 27.7 cm of acrylic, with 5.7 R/minute entry dose. The FD system reached the same 1.5-unit threshold at 32.2-cm attenuator thickness (16% greater), while delivering 10.8 R/minute (89% greater).

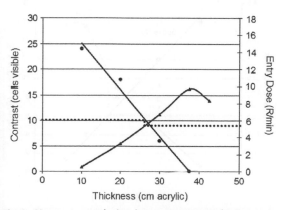
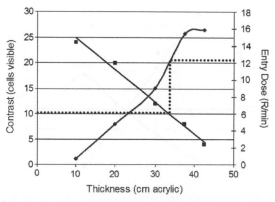

Fig. 3. Nomogram relating low-contrast resolution, x-ray dose, and attenuator thickness. Left panel: Image intensifier data. Circles represent contrast as a function of attenuator thickness, with regression line added ($y = -0.91x + 34.12$, $R^2 = 0.98$). Triangles represent x-ray entry dose. Ten units of image contrast corresponds to 26.6 cm of acrylic and 5.4 R/min entry dose. Right panel: Flat detector data. Squares represent contrast as a function of attenuator thickness, with regression line added ($y = -0.63x + 31.15$, $R^2 = 0.99$). Diamonds represent x-ray entry dose. Ten units of image contrast corresponds to 33.7 cm of acrylic and 12.1 R/minute entry dose.

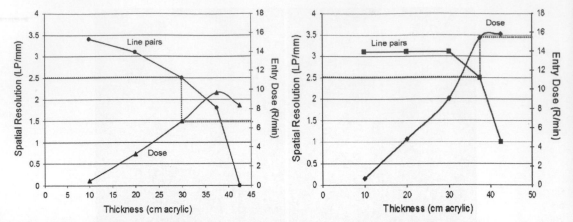

Fig. 4. Nomogram relating high-contrast spatial resolution, x-ray dose, and attenuator thickness. Left panel: Image intensifier data. Circles represent spatial resolution as a function of attenuator thickness, and triangles represent x-ray entry dose. Resolution of 2.5 LP/mm corresponds to 30 cm of acrylic and 6.7 R/min entry dose. Right panel: Flat detector data. Squares represent spatial resolution, and diamonds represent x-ray entry dose. Resolution of 3.1 LP/mm corresponds to 37.5 cm of acrylic and 15.5 R/min entry dose.

Overall Image Quality

At 30-cm thickness, II fluoroscopy delivered 21.8 units of image quality with a dose rate of 5.86 R/minute (**Fig. 6**). FD fluoroscopy reached the same 21.8-unit image quality threshold at 38-cm thickness, with a dose rate of 16.4 R/minute. To put this dose rate in perspective, an FD fluoroscopy procedure (without cine) would reach predicted limits for temporary skin injury at 12 minutes, and for permanent injury at 42 minutes.[3]

Cost of Image Quality

The radiation cost of image quality was similar for II and FD fluoroscopy (**Fig. 7**). The potentially higher

x-ray doses seen with FD fluoroscopy can be explained entirely by the ability of the FD system to generate useful images under challenging conditions of thick attenuators.

Acquisition Mode

Acquisition mode (or "cine") typically delivers 10 to 20 times the x-ray dose rate of fluoroscopy; it should be used sparingly for archive-quality angiography. However, when operators are faced with marginal image quality during interventional fluoroscopy, they sometimes obtain "cine runs" to help with critical decisions. As shown in **Fig. 8**, switching to a higher-dose fluoroscopy mode

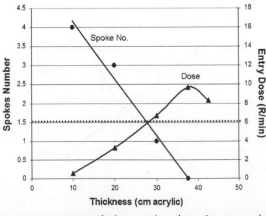
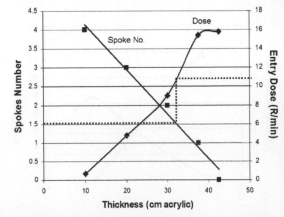

Fig. 5. Nomogram relating motion detection, x-ray dose, and attenuator thickness. Left panel: Image intensifier data. Circles represent spoke number as a function of attenuator thickness, with regression line added (y = −0.15x + 5.69, R^2 = 0.98). Triangles represent x-ray entry dose. A motion detection score of 1.5 corresponds to 27.7 cm of acrylic and 5.7 R/min entry dose. Right panel: Flat detector data. Squares represent contrast as a function of attenuator thickness, with regression line added (y = −0.12x + 5.34, R^2 = 0.98). Diamonds represent x-ray entry dose. A motion detection score of 1.5 corresponds to 32.2 cm of acrylic and 10.8 R/min entry dose.

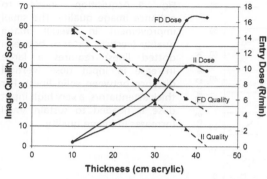

Fig. 6. Nomogram relating image quality score, x-ray dose, and attenuator thickness. Dashed lines are linear regression for image quality versus attenuator thickness. Squares are FD ($y = -1.29x + 72.6$, $R^2 = 0.98$), and triangles are II ($y = -1.8x + 75.1$, $R^2 = 0.99$). Solid lines represent dose as a function of detector thickness. Diamonds are FD and circles are II. Image quality and dose are similar for thin attenuators. For thick attenuators, FD provides superior image quality and higher x-ray doses.

(or to acquisition mode) did little to enhance II image quality. FD image quality, on the other hand, was substantially improved. As a result, FD systems may give operators of an incentive instinctively up-dose.

Although cine acquisitions can compensate for the loss of fluoroscopic image quality that occurs with heavy patients or steep projections, the modest gain in image quality is purchased with large increases in x-ray dose (**Fig. 9**).

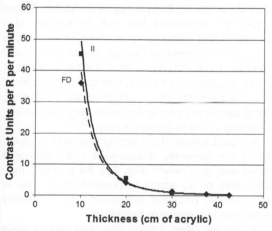

Fig. 7. Radiation cost of contrast resolution as a function of attenuator thickness. Squares represent II data, and solid line is regression curve ($y = 161,000x^{-3.51}$, $R^2 = 0.99$). Diamonds represent FD data, and dashed line is regression curve ($y = 82,000x^{-3.32}$, $R^2 = 0.99$). The radiation cost of contrast resolution is almost identical for II and FD fluoroscopy.

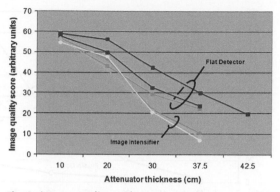

Fig. 8. Image quality and attenuator thickness. With thick attenuators, the II system obtained little benefit from higher x-ray doses (5 R/minute fluoro in light green, 10 R/minute fluoro in medium green, cine in dark green). The FD system was more likely to benefit from higher input doses (5 R/minute fluoro in pink, 10 R/minute fluoro in pink, cine in red).

A Danger Zone

Flat detectors, in combination with improved x-ray tubes, better generators, and stronger tables, have extended the working range of fluoroscopy (**Fig. 10**). It is now possible to work with very obese patients who require very high input doses—conditions that would not have been possible with older II-based systems.

CAPABILITY AND CONCERN: A CASE STUDY

The potential of FD fluoroscopy can be illustrated by a case study. A 475-pound man underwent emergency catheterization in a commercially available flat detector laboratory (Philips Allura FD-10, Best, Netherlands). Surprisingly good images were obtained, and the procedure was considered a success (**Fig. 11**). Before the procedure, two small squares of x-ray sensitive film were placed on the patient's chest wall to directly measure skin doses. In an effort to maximize image quality and minimize radiation exposure, all imaging was performed in the anterior-posterior projection, and a limited number of acquisitions were recorded (three left and one right coronary). The procedure was completed with a total exposure time of 5:43 minutes. Despite steps to minimize radiation dose during this abbreviated diagnostic procedure, the film indicated a skin entry dose of 3.0 Gy, which exceeded the 2.0 Gy threshold for early skin injury.

What if the operator had continued with an interventional procedure? Extrapolation of time and dose for this patient indicates that permanent skin injury would have occurred between 10 and

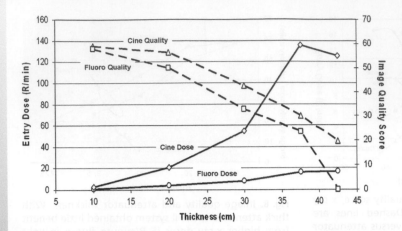

Fig. 9. Acquisition mode to enhance image quality. The small improvement in overall image quality (vertical distance between dotted lines) requires a large increase in input dose (vertical distance between solid lines). For thick attenuators, a very high input dose is needed to sustain small increases in image quality.

15 minutes, and serious skin necrosis would have occurred by 20 minutes.

MAKING THE CATH LAB SAFER
Understanding the Equipment

It is generally assumed that modern flat panel systems yield improved image quality with significant reductions in radiation dose, when compared with older image intensifier-based systems. The basis for this assumption is the improved detective quantum efficiency (DQE) and the greater dynamic range of the photodiode-based flat panel detector.[4–6] The higher DQE allows more of the x-ray photons passing through the patient to be captured and converted into image data (fewer wasted photons), whereas the greater dynamic range preserves usable contrast when few photons are available for image generation. This makes sense, but does it work in practice?

Studies of image quality and dose in digital radiography suggest that a 50% dose reduction is possible with FD technology;[4,6] however, little is known about patient exposure during FD

fluoroscopy.[7–9] The truth of the matter is that *new FD systems deliver almost the same dose per frame as older II-based systems*. This is because image quality is determined more by input dose than by the type of detector, and the trade-off between dose and quality is entirely a matter of personal preference. In most cases, dose is used to suppress the electronic noise that is inherent in digital flat detectors.[10]

Increasing Awareness

Although a decade has passed since the US Food and Drug Administration (FDA) Center for Devices and Radiological Health first issued its advisory warning to health care institutions about the risk of radiation burns from fluoroscopy,[11] injuries continue to occur in increasing numbers.[12–17] Federal regulations governing the maximum allowable dose rate for fluoroscopy in the United States have not eliminated the risk of serious skin burns.[18] And although prominent organizations such as the American College of Cardiology and the FDA have long recognized the seriousness of x-ray exposure in the catheterization laboratory and the need for structured physician education, most practicing physicians have very little understanding of the radiological risks.[19–21]

A recent survey at our facility showed that operators are generally unaware of x-ray exposure rates and skin doses (**Fig. 12**). As a result, they take little or no action to prevent injury. This is unfortunate, because skin dose can be greatly influenced by operator technique.

A graphic dose display can help cardiologists choose gantry angles, table heights, and other parameters that minimize radiation exposure (**Fig. 13**). It replaces the difficult terminology of radiation physics with a simple "speedometer" for dose rate and a "fuel gauge" for accumulated skin dose. A "safe working time" prediction allows

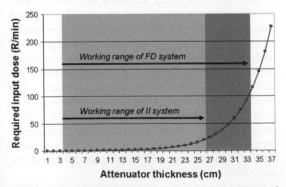

Fig. 10. Flat detectors extend the working range of fluoroscopy into a zone of high x-ray doses. Shaded areas indicate the range of tissue thickness likely to be encountered in clinical practice.

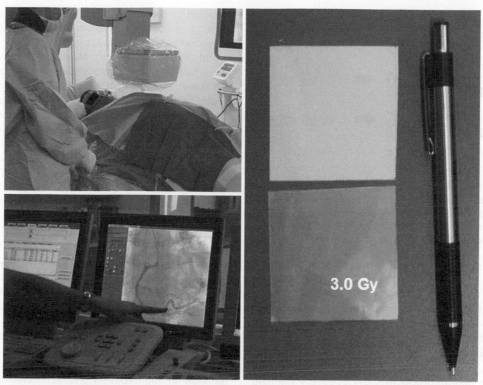

Fig. 11. Case study. This obese patient was successfully imaged (*left*), but accumulated a 3.0-Gy skin dose in less than 6 minutes. The threshold for injury to healthy skin is about 2.0 Gy. Skin dose was measured directly with radiochromic film (*right*).

operators to budget their time or to modify their technique as necessary. Because the display responds in real time to operator adjustments, it encourages simple steps that can dramatically reduce x-ray doses. This helps operators learn to use fluoroscopy safely. The display also alerts the operator when any skin zone has received a safe dose limit of 2.0 Gy, reducing the risk of unintended injury.

NEW METHODS FOR NEW EQUIPMENT
Steps to Optimize Quality

Flat detectors are frequently operated using techniques that were developed for image intensifiers.

For decades, cardiac angiographers were taught to use high magnifications and to pan the table to keep vessels centered. This was done because image intensifiers provided their best spatial resolution in the central portion of the image and at high magnification, and because the curved face of the intensifier caused pincushion distortion at the periphery. In addition, the limited grayscale resolution of image intensifiers often caused "white-outs" around the edges of the image.

Flat detectors do not suffer from any of these limitations. The spatial resolution of a flat detector is uniform from edge-to-edge, and is determined

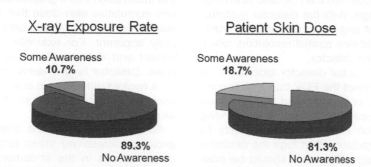

Fig. 12. Survey of dose awareness in one catheterization laboratory. Sampling included 100 unselected procedures. Most operators are unaware of x-ray exposure rates or skin doses.

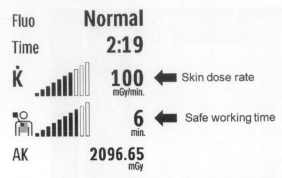

Fluo   **Normal**

Time   **2:19**

K̇ ▁▂▃▄▅▆▊   **100** ← Skin dose rate
                mGy/min.

👤 ▁▂▃▄▅▆▊   **6** ← Safe working time
                min.

AK   **2096.65**
                mGy

Fig. 13. Real-time dose awareness. This indicates skin dose rate, accumulated skin dose by body region, and the safe working time remaining in any given projection. The values change in real time whenever the operator adjusts angle, table height, detector height, frame rate, or any other parameter that affects dose rate.

by the size of the elements in the detector matrix, not by the degree of magnification. There is no pincushion distortion. The wide dynamic range gives the entire image a usable grayscale.

With flat detectors, panning and magnification can be counterproductive. Unnecessary panning introduces motion artifacts and interferes with digital noise suppression algorithms. Magnification always requires higher x-ray dose rates. Image intensifiers need increased doses to maintain image brightness when less of the detector face is exposed. Because dose rate is inversely proportional to detector area, a 6-cm field of view (FOV) (36 cm²) requires nearly twice the dose rate of an 8-cm FOV (64 cm²). Flat detectors do not have this problem, but smaller FOVs still require higher dose rates. Flat detectors use dose to suppress noise, which is visually more apparent on magnified images. Dose increases of 50% to 100% can occur with each reduction in field size. Excessive magnification can unexpectedly degrade image quality. This happens when the dose increase is provided by a longer pulse width, which blurs moving structures. Electronic zoom can then be used to enlarge the displayed image. With flat detector systems, the combination of larger field size and electronic zoom does not sacrifice spatial resolution, which is determined by the detector.

When working in a flat detector laboratory, an operator should select the FOV that just encompasses the region of interest, and then collimate to avoid unnecessary exposure of surrounding tissues. Collimation improves image quality by reducing scatter radiation that fogs the desirable portion of the image. The table should be positioned before acquisition, and then panned as little as possible. In most cases, panning is not

necessary. When panning is required, as for viewing of collateral vessels, the table should be moved slowly and deliberately.

Flat detectors are uniquely capable of supporting advanced image processing techniques that will make catheterization faster and safer. Diagnostic tools that create CT-like images from rotational acquisitions will depict soft tissues and provide 3D planning for interventional procedures. Navigational tools that fuse live fluoroscopy with 3D reconstructions of the vessel tree will guide operators through tortuous vasculature. Through improved planning and improved visualization, these features will minimize the use of radiation during complex interventions.

Steps to Minimize Risk

Radiation safety is more important now than ever before. Patient skin injuries are inexcusable because they do not occur at x-ray doses below a safe threshold, and modern FD systems provide all the information that an operator needs to manage the dose that is delivered. Recent studies have found significant (and permanent) DNA damage in high-volume interventional cardiologists.[22,23] Physicians must be able to understand their equipment well enough to protect their patients and themselves.

It might seem that modern FD fluoroscopy systems require very little input from the operator. In fact, most of the determinants of x-ray dose are under the operator's control. Table height, detector height, frame rate, mode, viewing angle, and beam-on time are all major determinants of dose. All are chosen by the operator. Newer FD fluoroscopy systems help the operator understand how these parameters affect dose. They also incorporate many dose-saving features that can greatly improve safety.

Newer FD fluoroscopy systems track radiation output along with table height, gantry angle, and detector height. As we have seen, they can convert this information into a graphic display of dose rate and cumulative skin dose that is easy to understand. Actions that reduce exposure are immediately apparent. For example, the gap between patient and detector is a major determinant of dose. Detector height alone can be responsible for a twofold difference in dose rate. The detector should always be placed as close to the patient as possible.

Small adjustments that affect beam path—avoiding excessively steep angles and avoiding dense tissues in the abdomen and spine—can dramatically reduce dose. In most cases, large portions of an interventional procedure can be

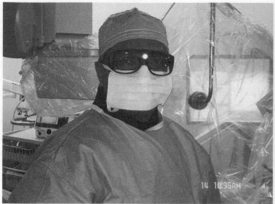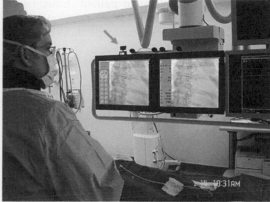

Fig. 14. Automatic fluoroscopy lockout. A reflector (*left panel*) is tracked by a small infrared camera (*arrow*). The system stops x-ray production whenever the operator looks away from the monitor.

performed in shallow projections that minimize dose. Steep angles can be used briefly to position stents and define branch points.

Newer FD systems usually provide several fluoroscopy modes, each with a different balance between image quality and dose. The "low-dose fluoro" setting typically delivers half the dose rate of "normal fluoro" and is suitable for positioning diagnostic catheters, electrophysiology catheters, and pacing leads.

Some FD systems can archive and replay fluoroscopy. Stored fluoroscopy clips are usually adequate to guide the placement of interventional hardware and to identify femoral puncture sites. Fluoroscopy clips require less than one-tenth the dose of acquisitions, which can be reserved for diagnostic angiography and final documentation after interventions.

Radiation doses can also be minimized by selecting the lowest frame rate appropriate for the task. For coronary work, 15 fps acquisitions are usually necessary, but for extremities 1 fps may be adequate. Newer systems offer a variety of low frame rate protocols, such as 7.5 fps fluoroscopy for electrophysiology procedures, and

single-frame acquisitions to document the position of hardware.

A skilled operator can greatly extend the safe working time through a combination of dose-saving measures such as rationing the use of steep projections, spreading the dose over several different projections, and limiting acquisitions. In the near future, FD laboratories will add smart dose displays and real-time personal dose monitors that provide immediate feedback and suggest ways to minimize the risks of radiation. They may even take an active role. For example, a smart system can eliminate unnecessary x-ray exposure by automatically disabling the foot switch whenever an operator looks away from the live monitor (**Fig. 14**). This prototype system is based on a miniature infrared camera that tracks the operator's head. We have found that 15% of the fluoroscopy time during general cath lab procedures is unnecessary because it occurs when the operator is not viewing an image (**Fig. 15**).

SUMMARY

Flat detector fluoroscopy systems provide new capabilities and new hazards. We have seen how the combination of enhanced detector performance and automatic exposure control can allow operators to deliver large doses of radiation to the skin during procedures that involve heavy patients or steep projections. Cardiologists must respect these powerful systems and learn how to operate them safely. They should avoid steep projections during prolonged procedures, and they should resist the temptation to use high-dose cine acquisitions to supplement fluoroscopy during interventional procedures. They should understand that fluoroscopy time is a poor measure of radiation risk because dose rates can

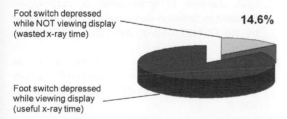

Foot switch depressed while NOT viewing display (wasted x-ray time) — **14.6%**

Foot switch depressed while viewing display (useful x-ray time)

Fig. 15. Unnecessary radiation. In a general cath lab setting, 15% of the total fluoroscopy time occurs when operators are not viewing the image. This fraction constitutes unnecessary radiation exposure that can be eliminated.

vary greatly from patient to patient. Equipment manufacturers must continue to develop user-friendly displays that encourage operators to apply dose-saving features.

For each additional centimeter of tissue penetrated, the input dose must be increased by approximately 25%. Adding 3 cm of tissue thickness requires twice the input dose. Adding 8 cm of tissue requires a sixfold dose increase.

REFERENCES

1. National Electrical Manufacturers Association. Characteristics of and test procedures for a phantom to benchmark cardiac fluoroscopic and photographic performance: Proceedings of the National Electrical Manufacturers Association; 2000. NEMA Standards Publication #XR21-2000.
2. Chambers CE, Phillips WJ, Cowley MJ, Laboratory Performance Standards Committee; Society for cardiac angiography and interventions. Image quality assessment and the NEMA/SCA&I phantom. Catheter Cardiovasc Interv 2001;52(1):73.
3. Wagner LK, Eifel PJ, Geise RA. Potential biological effects following high x-ray dose interventional procedures. J Vasc Interv Radiol 1994;5:71–84.
4. Spahn M, Strotzer M, Völk M, et al. Digital radiography with a large-area, amorphous-silicon, flat-panel X-ray detector system. Invest Radiol 2000;35:260–6.
5. Neitzel U, Böhm A, Maack I. Comparison of low-contrast detail detectability with five different conventional and digital radiographic imaging systems. In: Krupinski EA, editor. Proceedings of the SPIE. San Diego (CA); 2007. p. 216–23.
6. Geijer H, Beckman KW, Andersson T, et al. Image quality vs radiation dose for a flat-panel amorphous silicon detector: a phantom study. Eur Radiol 2001; 11:1704–9.
7. Tsapaki V, Kottou S, Kollaros N, et al. Dose performance evaluation of a charge coupled device and a flat-panel digital fluoroscopy system recently installed in an interventional cardiology laboratory. Radiat Prot Dosimetry 2004;111(3):297–304.
8. Maolinbay M, El-Mohri Y, Antonuk LE, et al. Additive noise properties of active matrix flat-panel imagers. Med Phys 2000;27:1841–54.
9. Tsapaki V, Kottou S, Kollaros N, et al. Comparison of a conventional and a flat-panel digital system in interventional cardiology. Br J Radiol 2004;77(919):562–7.
10. Marshall NW, Kotre CJ, Robson KJ, et al. Receptor dose in digital fluorography: a comparison between theory and practice. Phys Med Biol 2001;46(4):1283–96.
11. US Department of Health. FDA Public Health Advisory: Avoidance of serious x-ray-induced skin injuries to patients during fluoroscopically-guided procedures. Available at: http://www.fda.gov/MedicalDevices/Safety/AlertsandNotices/PublicHealthNotifications/ucm063084.htm. Accessed September 9,1994.
12. Shope TB. Radiation-induced skin injuries from fluoroscopy. Radiographics 1996;16(5):1195–9.
13. Rosenthal LS, Beck TJ, Williams J, et al. Acute radiation dermatitis following radiofrequency catheter ablation of atrioventricular nodal reentrant tachycardia. Pacing Clin Electrophysiol 1997;20(7): 1834–9.
14. Sovik E, Klow NE, Hellesnes J, et al. Radiation-induced skin injury after percutaneous transluminal coronary angioplasty. Case report. Acta Radiol 1996;37(3 Pt 1):305–6.
15. Lichtenstein DA, Klapholz L, Vardy DA, et al. Chronic radiodermatitis following cardiac catheterization. Arch Dermatol 1996;132(6):663–7.
16. Knautz MA, Abele DC, Reynolds TL. Radiodermatitis after transjugular intrahepatic portosystemic shunt. South Med J 1997;90(3):352–6.
17. Nahass GT. Acute radiodermatitis after radiofrequency catheter ablation. J Am Acad Dermatol 1997;36(5 Pt 2):881–4.
18. US Department of Health and Human Services. Federal performance standard for diagnostic x-ray systems and their major components. USFDA; 1994. Fed Regist 1993;58(83):26386–406.
19. Brinker JA. Use of radiographic devices by cardiologists. American College of Cardiology Cardiac Catheterization Committee. J Am Coll Cardiol 1995;25(7):1738–9.
20. Limacher MC, Douglas PS, Germano G, et al. ACC expert consensus document. Radiation safety in the practice of cardiology. American College of Cardiology. J Am Coll Cardiol 1998;31(4):892–913 [review].
21. Radiation injuries and fluoroscopy, United States Food and Drug Administration. Center for Devices and Radiological Health. Available at: http://www.fda.gov/cdrh/radinj.html. Accessed April 6, 2009.
22. Boyaci B, Yalcin R, Cengel A, et al. Evaluation of DNA damage in lymphocytes of cardiologists exposed to radiation during cardiac catheterization by the COMET ASSAY. Jpn Heart J 2004;45(5): 845–53.
23. Andreassi MG, Cioppa A, Botto N, et al. Somatic DNA damage in interventional cardiologists: a case-control study. FASEB J 2005;19(8): 998–9.

Rotational Coronary Angiography

Andrew J.P. Klein, MD[a],*, Joel A. Garcia, MD[b,c]

KEYWORDS

- Angiography • Coronary • Standard angiography
- Rotational angiography • Dual axis
- Off-axis rotation • 180° rotation

Catheter-based coronary angiography is the gold standard for the diagnosis of coronary artery disease (CAD), which is the leading cause of mortality worldwide. Despite its widespread use in the diagnosis and treatment of atherosclerotic disease, the imaging characteristics of angiography "may misrepresent, impair, or alter the accurate representation of vascular structures."[1] Discrepancies between coronary angiography and intravascular ultrasound,[2,3] angioscopy,[4–6] physiologic flow measurements,[7–9] and autopsy[10–12] have further underscored angiography's limitations.[13] These discrepancies are most evident in the presence of eccentric or complicated lesions,[10,11,14] where the shortcomings of angiography have been ascribed to its luminology dataset.[15]

One explanation for the diagnostic inaccuracy of angiography has been the use of relatively few static or fixed acquisitions that are obtained during standard angiography (SA). In fact, these angiographic acquisitions are operator-dependent, based on heuristic experience, and are limited by time, safety, and cost. Most operators obtain between four and six views of the left coronary tree and two to three views of the right coronary tree in an attempt to overcome vessel foreshortening, overlap, and minimize any potential underestimation of vessel tortuosity.[15–18] The resulting gap, however, between the acquired adjacent projections, and thus the potential deviation from the optimal angle of observation, has been noted to range from 30° to greater than 90° when only

two projections are used, which can lead to a gross underestimation of lesion severity.[13,19]

In an effort to overcome the numerous limitations of standard coronary angiography, Tommasini and colleagues[19] in 1998 first advanced the clinical use of "panoramic coronary angiography," which later became known as rotational angiography (RA). This new technique employed the manual movement of the gantry through a series of four 25° arcs, two in the cranial and caudal positions, respectively. In this landmark article, Tommasini reported that via RA, almost 25% of patients had critical lesions, which were clearly missed with conventional angiography but evident on panoramic angiography. The investigators concluded that RA, by providing operators with numerous dynamic images, instead of the standard static six to eight, enhanced diagnostic accuracy. Furthermore, this group reported a reduction in contrast and cine time with this new technique: the first suggestion that, indeed, RA may not only be better in terms of diagnostic capability, but also safer than conventional SA.

In the last decade, advances in technology have permitted an automation of the rotational acquisition process, such that now RA is commercially available on a number of X-ray systems. Given the new automated ability to obtain numerous images in one acquisition, several investigators have evaluated the safety and efficacy of RA compared to conventional angiography. The first prospective, randomized study comparing these

[a] Division of Cardiology, Department of Medicine, John Cochran Veterans Affairs Medical Center, 915 N. Grand Blvd. St. Louis, MO 63104, USA
[b] University of Colorado Health Sciences Center, Denver, CO, USA
[c] Division of Cardiology, Denver Health Medical Center, 777 Bannock Street, Mail Code 0960. Denver, CO 80204, USA
* Corresponding author.
E-mail addresses: andrew.klein@ucdenver.edu; ajpkmd@hotmail.com (A.J.P. Klein).

Cardiol Clin 27 (2009) 395–405
doi:10.1016/j.ccl.2009.03.002
0733-8651/09/$ – see front matter © 2009 Elsevier Inc. All rights reserved.

cardiology.theclinics.com

two modalities was performed in 2004.[20] Numerous other studies examined how RA compares to SA with respect to contrast use, radiation exposure, and procedural time followed. Though these studies are reviewed in detail later in this article, in summary, RA has consistently been shown to decrease contrast use and potentially radiation exposure to both the patient and the operator. Given the direct relationship between contrast volume, the risk of contrast-induced nephropathy (CIN) and the as low as reasonably achievable radiation-dose principle, these features of RA make it the preferred angiographic acquisition method.

Given the mortality associated with CAD and the numerous limitations of SA, the imperative need for the optimization of the safety, sensitivity, and specificity of this critical procedure cannot be underestimated. RA has represented a revolutionary development toward the enhancement of this invasive procedure. This article examines the development of RA from its first theoretical conception in 1983[18] to the most recent revolutionary concept of dual-axis rotational angiography (DARCA). RA's advantages and disadvantages, technique, and research applications are also reviewed.

SINGLE-AXIS ROTATIONAL CORONARY ANGIOGRAPHY

The first developed and most commonly used type of RA is single-axis rotational angiography. This concept was born from the idea that a large number of views are required to eliminate the potential error associated with a diameter assessment of highly elliptical lumen (ie, the coronary artery).[18] Single-axis RA acquires the same images and several more as traditional angiography, but is automated, can be standardized, and provides an extensive panoramic view of key anatomic features for diagnostic and interventional purposes.

Single-axis rotational coronary angiography by definition is an image acquisition on the same or similar angulation planes (cranial, postero-anterior, or caudal) that extends from right anterior oblique (RAO) to left anterior oblique (LAO) or vice versa. Keeping the acquisition on the same plane requires that, for a complete coronary evaluation, the alternate plane is imaged in an effort to obtain orthogonal views, which have been shown to decrease error estimating coronary cross-sectional diameters.[18] For this reason a complete rotational evaluation will consist of a cranial (Fig. 1A and Video 1a) (All videos can be accessed in the online version of this article at: http://www.cardiology.theclinics. com/) and a caudal rotation of 120° for the left coronary arterial system (LCA) (Fig. 1B and Video 1b) and a cranial rotation of 120° for the right coronary artery (RCA) (Fig. 2 and Video 2). While some imaging systems commercially available can perform cranial and caudal rotations, some others are limited to a rotation with no angulation in the postero-anterior (PA) plane.

Continuous display of images through RA immediately provides the operator a survey or

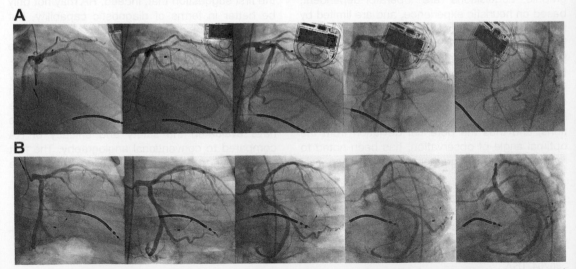

Fig. 1. (A) Rotational coronary angiography of the left coronary artery extending from 60° RAO to 60° LAO with a cranial angulation. The patient has a dual-chamber pacemaker and defibrillator coil that presents an additional challenge to the selection of adequate angiographic views. (B) Rotational coronary angiography of the left coronary artery (LCA) extending from 60° RAO to 60° left anterior oblique (LAO) with a caudal angulation.

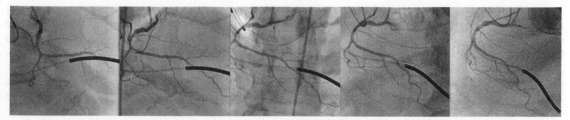

Fig. 2. Same patient as in **Fig. 1** *A* and *B* with challenging imaging. Rotational coronary angiography of the right coronary artery (RAO) extending from 60° right anterior oblique (RAO) to 60° left anterior oblique (LAO) with a cranial angulation.

three-dimensional (3D)-like image of the coronary tree. RA also permits the modeling of coronary arteries through specific software. This modeling can then be used to evaluate the various standard views that are obtained during SA with respect to vessel foreshortening and overlap in an attempt to overcome these limitations. Another major difference between both image acquisitions is that RA provides a large amount of information regarding the coronary tree. A complete coronary evaluation using RA provides up to 360 projections (three acquisitions of 120 frames each) of the arterial tree from different angles, as opposed to the limited views provided by SA. The review of RA images is relatively easy once the operator becomes accustomed to the sweeping motion of the coronary tree. In the authors' experience with cardiology fellows, a relatively few number of RA angiograms is required before one becomes used to identifying all vessels and lesions.

RA Technique

Isocentering

For the most part, setting up for a rotational run is straight forward and simple. The critical initial procedural step before performing RA is isocentering. As noted in one study, the need for additional static-angiographic projections, which thus decreases the power of RA, is most often because of improper isocentering.[21] The field of view (FOV) must first be selected and the appropriate FOV is dictated by the heart size, though most acquisitions can be performed on either 8-inch or at least less than a 12-inch FOV. In the authors' laboratory, a 10.5-inch FOV is used when the 8-inch FOV is not large enough. After isocentering the heart in PA by table panning, the gantry is then moved to the lateral position (60 degrees LAO) where, by elevating or lowering the table, the heart is isocentered (no lateral table movement should be performed in this stage).

Rotational scan set-up

Once the heart is isocentered (ideally with a < 10.5-inch FOV), the operator must ensure that the X-ray system setting is set to rotational mode. In most commercially available systems, cranial and caudal rotational rolls are available. Once in the proper mode, depending upon the system, the operator most often only needs to press the blinking end-position button, which will become a solid light once the predetermined position is reached. This is followed by holding down the blinking begin-position button, which will also become a solid light once the predetermined position is reached. The gantry should automatically sweep the predetermined arc in a safety mode, looking for potential hazards that would cause a collision, such as the patient's arms, intravenous tubing, or other hazards. Once cleared, the system is ready to acquire the rotational image. At this point, activating the acquisition pedal will result in an automatic sweeping movement of the gantry that will generate numerous images (Video 3). These images cannot be simply substituted by a nonisocentered operator-driven motion of the gantry, as it results in a nonstandardized or nonreproducible acquisition. The sweeping arc is completed in approximately 4 seconds, which needs to be taken into account for the necessary set-up of the contrast injection during the run. Most operators who perform RA rely on a power-injection system to ensure complete vessel opacification, though this is not absolutely mandatory. Once the acquisition starts, contrast is injected to avoid losing necessary information in the run. The injection of contrast prior to the image acquisition technique can limit the evaluation of thrombosis in myocardial infarction (TIMI) flow. If TIMI flow or vessel calcification is desired, one can add a 0.5- to 0.8-second delay at the beginning of the acquisition to allow for the evaluation of flow before the rotation starts. This upgraded acquisition arc will take around 5.2 seconds to be completed and allows for a more superior evaluation. Likewise, a delay at the end of the acquisition can be added to permit the evaluation of collateral circulation. All single-axis acquisitions (not extended acquisitions) can be completed with either a standard 12-mL manifold or an automated injector.

Advantages in Using RA

Contrast use

One potential complication of coronary angiography that is associated with increased morbidity and mortality is CIN. The risk of CIN is associated with numerous factors, including increased contrast volume.[22] Angiographic techniques that limit contrast use may therefore improve patient safety.[21] Several studies have compared the contrast utilization in RA and SA.[19–21,23,24] Though differences exist between these studies, RA has been shown to consistently reduce contrast use. These studies have shown a decrease between 19%-61%, with the most recent flat-detector study showing a 40% reduction,[21] and should therefore theoretically decrease the risk of CIN.

Radiation exposure

The same studies that compared contrast use also investigated RA's impact on radiation exposure.[19–21,23,24] While differences exist between studies in terms of the use of image intensifiers versus flat-panel detectors, and the inclusion of operators with varying degrees of experience in RA, the common denominator has been a decrease or no significant difference in radiation exposure when RA is compared with SA. The first randomized, controlled safety study by Maddox and colleagues,[20] which used an older angiographic system with an image intensifier (Philips Integris Allura), was specifically designed to answer this question of radiation exposure. This study found a statistically significant 28% reduction in radiation exposure. In addition, this study was the only one that examined primary and secondary operator-effective dose equivalents. RA again showed a significant difference in radiation exposure to both operators when compared with SA. Given a potential lifetime of radiation exposure and its stochastic effects, even a small decrease may be clinically significant. A more recent study, which used a flat-panel detector, showed no difference in radiation exposure[21] for both SA and RA, but a significant decrease in radiation was seen when compared with the image-intensifier reported exposure in the safety study.[20] It should be noted that RA uses 30 frames per second compared with the standard 15 frames per second, and that the source-to-image distance is often much higher during RA (to

accommodate for the rotation). All of these factors should increase the amount of radiation, not decrease it. However, the decrease in the total amount of images acquired in a RA study is the driving mechanism for the reduction. Regardless, the use of RA either reduces or has a neutral effect upon radiation exposure, both to the patients and to the operators.

Procedural time

Of the major studies investigating the impact of RA, two have also examined procedural time. These studies revealed that the use of RA did, at the minimum, result in an increase in procedural time. In fact, one study demonstrated a decrease in procedural time[20] while the other showed no significant change in this variable.[21] It is, however, important to note that each of these studies employed operators with varying degrees of RA experience and that there is an obvious learning curve when learning how to isocenter. A subsequent image-content evaluation of RA has shown a further decrease in procedural time when compared with prior evaluations, showing that conquering the learning curve results in improved timing.[25] In addition, X-ray systems have become faster and more user friendly, allowing for a more efficient preparation of the rotational runs.

Screening adequacy and lesion assessment

Quantitative and qualitative lesion assessment is a pivotal part of coronary angiography. RA has the power to detect a similar or higher amount of lesions when directly compared with SA.[19,24] Ongoing studies show very promising results that establish the noninferiority—and in some instances superiority—of the image content in RA when compared with SA. The authors' group has shown that despite the larger FOV, the use of quantitative coronary angiography (QCA) measurements is no different when comparing RA and SA.[25] This has been the product of an image-content evaluation comparing RA to SA. RA is comparable and in some instances superior to SA in the lesion assessment, diagnostic screening adequacy, and QCA evaluation of patients undergoing diagnostic angiography.[25] Thus, it is believed that RA can replace SA in the diagnosis of CAD, given its image-content properties.

Limitations

Despite the visual appeal, better safety, and the standardized acquisition technique of RA, the inherent limitations of 2D-projection imaging remain. It is important to note that the evaluation of RA acquisitions can be easily mastered with little experience. While RA may improve the ability to visualize a lesion, the accurate selection of the optimal projection is still dependent upon the operator's visual skills. Furthermore, RA cannot simulate views based on acquired images and provides no quantification of important 3D-vessel features.

RA can be performed in most patients; however, individuals with significant abdominal girth may make the positioning of the gantry difficult. In such patients, often truncation of the rotation (ie, less LAO–RAO acquisition angles) is required. While isocentering can be easily mastered, it is the most common limitation in the adoption of RA, as a learning curve does exist. RA is a reasonably new technology provided by multiple vendors but may not be available in older imaging systems. While it can be adapted to any laboratory, the use of RA is mostly limited by the inability of acquiring newer systems that provide this technology.

Extended Rotational (or 180° Rotation) Coronary Angiography

Despite the 3D perspective provided by RA, 2D limitations still exist, including the inability to provide 3D-volumetric vessel features. There has been, however, an evolution of technology that has permitted the generation of newer and revolutionary acquisition arcs designed to provide enough angiographic information that could be processed as volumetric "computed tomography-like" data.

Single-axis extended rotational coronary angiography, or the 180° rotation, is the product of an effort to convert the X-ray based angiographic projection information into volumetric data.

Because of all the limitations to which angiography is exposed (ie, cardiac motion, respiratory movement), converting this data requires a longer RA acquisition. This long acquisition will ideally permit gated reconstruction of angiograms, respiratory motion compensation, or more recently iterative reconstructions.[26]

The traditional single-axis rotation goes from 55° to 60° of RAO to 55° to 60° LAO, either cranial or caudal. The 180° acquisition goes from 120° LAO to 60° RAO with no angulation (**Fig. 3** and Video 4). This longer imaging allows for the reconstruction of the vessel in a volumetric fashion, but clearly uses a longer arc sweep, requiring more time and subsequently a longer contrast injection. As first mentioned by Tommasini,[19] longer coronary injections must be handled carefully given the arrythmogenic effects of contrast. The safety of a longer contrast injection (< 7.1 seconds) has been evaluated with no significant hemodynamic effects.[27] The reader should note that Iodixanol was the only contrast used during this safety study and that such an injection protocol is not yet tested in patients with unstable coronary syndromes. Additionally, the authors suggest that contrast volumes and duration do not exceed that evaluated by the study.

180° RA technique

The set up of the 180° rotation is very similar to that of the single-axis rotation already described. Isocentering and positioning the gantry is identical to the single-axis rotation. The only difference is that the rotation of the gantry is extended to cover

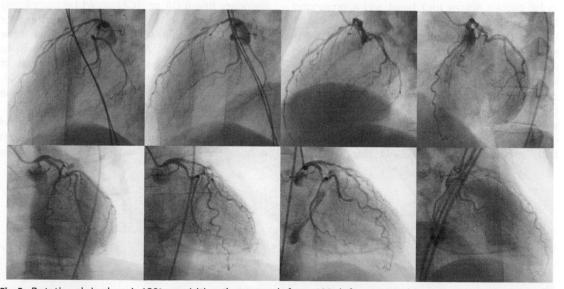

Fig. 3. Rotational single-axis 180° acquisition that extends from 120° left anterior oblique (LAO) to 60° right anterior oblique (RAO).

a wider arc (120° LAO° to 60° RAO). These changes result in several limitations outlined below:

1. The patient is required to be able to lift his arms above the head to avoid the gantry to clear the 90° angle in LAO.
2. The patient is also required to hold his breath in end-expiration for the duration of the acquisition to minimize respiratory motion (approximately 7 seconds).
3. A wider FOV is used (often 10.5 to 13 inches).

Advantages

The main arena wherein the 180° rotation has been used is in research for the purpose of 3D-coronary vessel-gated reconstructions. While the 180° rotation has been instrumental in research, its image content and clinical value had not been evaluated until recently. Preliminary data from the authors' laboratory shows that the 180° rotation results in clinically meaningful images for screening adequacy and lesion assessment. As the 180° acquisition is performed only once for the left coronary system, in place of the usual RA cranial and caudal roll, it may result in a decrease in total radiation exposure and contrast volume use. A more rigorous safety study that compares the 180° rotation to SA is necessary.

Limitations

The acquisition of this 180° rotation requires expertise in isocentering to allow the gantry to clear the steep angles used (120° LAO), and there is a clear learning curve for even experienced RA operators. Given the need for the patient's arms to be placed above their head and a prolonged breath-hold, this type of acquisition can be challenging to some patients. Additionally, given the steep LAO position, there may be an increase in radiation to the primary operator. While the safety of the longer injection has been proven, the value of the resulting angiogram needs to be more rigorously evaluated. Further studies are required that evaluate the clinical usefulness of the 2D 180° rotation and the subsequent coronary reconstruction, and its impact on CAD diagnosis and subsequent interventions. This is especially important, as the image content evaluation of the single-axis rotation has not included an evaluation where no angulation was used, as it is the case of the 180° rotation. Therefore, the results of this image-content study should not be extrapolated to the 180° degree technique.

DUAL-AXIS ROTATIONAL CORONARY ANGIOGRAPHY

The advent of RA in 1997 represented a huge leap in coronary angiography and imaging science. With numerous studies showing its improved safety profile and enhanced diagnostic capabilities, it is surprising that RA is not more widely used in catheterization suites. Advances in imaging technology and gantry rotational speeds have now permitted the next large step in the evolution of RA: dual-axis rotational coronary angiography (DARCA) (X-perSwing™ Philips Health care, Best, The Netherlands).

DARCA, which is a type of RA with simultaneous cranial-to-caudal and LAO-to-RAO acquisition arcs (**Fig. 4** and Videos 5 and 6), was built from two similar but distinct concepts. The first concept is the cornerstone principle that traditional left coronary angiography (LCA) typically involves the use of cranial and caudal angulation in addition to LAO and RAO gantry positions. This fact led to the standard RA practice of performing two rotational acquisitions of the LCA (cranial and caudal) and one cranial acquisition of the right coronary artery (RCA). If one acquisition encompasses all of the aforementioned regions, each coronary tree (LCA or RCA) could be completely evaluated using only one coronary injection for a total of two acquisitions, instead of the three with single-axis RA. As RA has been shown to decrease contrast use and radiation and has at least a neutral effect on procedural time, an acquisition that further shortens the number of runs should prove to be superior.

DARCA was also generated from the second concept that any rotational acquisition must encompass clinically useful and efficacious

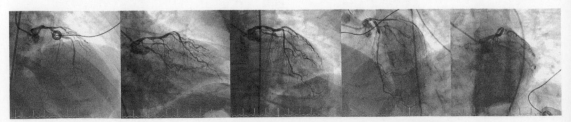

Fig. 4. A few selected frames of Dual-axis (RA) rotational coronary angiography (DARCA).

projection angles. The exact pathway that the gantry follows in DARCA was not randomly chosen. The DARCA gantry pathway was first fabricated from the same gantry arc acquisitions that are present in standard RA, with a simple connection arc placed between the cranial and caudal rolls. Thus, the projection angles assessed during DARCA easily encompass the standard gantry positions—that is, the four corners—and more by combining both the cranial and caudal projection during one single acquisition. The most recent and commercially available gantry pathway of DARCA is even more scientifically based. Using 3D models generated from RA, the authors[28] investigated the various degrees of fore-shortening and overlap seen during angiography for all first- and second-order coronary vessels. Using this data, the gantry pathway for DARCA was further enhanced such that it would permit visualization of all parts of the coronary tree, with minimization of vessel overlap and foreshortening.

DARCA Rotational Technique

Isocentering
The technique required for DARCA does not differ from single-axis RA. Isocentering is critical and is performed in the same aforementioned fashion. The FOV chosen can usually be less than 13 inches and often the entire acquisition is able to be obtained on 10.5 inches or 8 inches, thus providing operators similar image magnification as static SA.

In contrast to the 180° rotation, the patient may leave their arms at their side for DARCA, which enhances its ease of use. The gantry rotation is preset and simply requires following the same procedure as for single-axis RA. The length of the acquisition varies by coronary tree. Typically for the LCA, there is a less than 6.5-second acquisition and for the RCA, a less than 3.5-second acquisition. As prolonged coronary injections have been previously shown to be safe,[27] there should be no adverse effects from these types of injections. In fact, in the authors' preliminary experience with DARCA, neither adverse events nor any significant hemodynamic perturbations with these prolonged coronary injections were seen. Given the duration of the injection, a power injection system is recommended. Typically, the authors have been able to fill the LCA tree using a set rate of 2.0 cc to 2.5 cc per second for a total of 18 cc (not to be exceeded) of contrast. Iodixanol has been the only contrast agent used for DARCA in the authors' laboratory, given it is the only one studied and confirmed to be safe in prolonged injections.[27] As the RCA is a shorter acquisition, the authors have used a rate of 1.5 cc to 2 cc

per second for a total of 10 cc of contrast. With the authors' specific power injection system (ACIST, Acist Medical Systems, Eden Prairie, Minnesota), it is possible to synchronize the coronary injection with the image acquisition to opacify all vessels during all frames. A delay of 0.5 seconds could also be entered to evaluate TIMI flow or vessel calcification according to operator preference. Overall, a complete evaluation of the coronary tree can often be accomplished with less than 30 cc of contrast.

Advantages
DARCA has only been commercially available since September of 2008, and thus no current studies are published regarding the safety and efficacy of this revolutionary type of imaging. Preliminary data from the authors' laboratory in a pilot study of 15 patients undergoing both SA and DARCA (using a flat-panel detector) show a 47% reduction in contrast use, a 38% reduction in patient-delivered radiation, and a 28% reduction in procedural time.[29] With respect to image quality, data from the authors' pilot study has shown that operators feel that the images from DARCA are noninferior, if not superior, to those obtained during SA. Clearly, larger studies evaluating the safety and efficacy of DARCA are required.

Limitations
As with the 180° rotation, the gantry must rotate through a number of projection angles. Therefore, it is imperative that all potential collisions be removed before performing DARCA, given the dual-axis movement of the gantry arm. Given the cranial-to-caudal movement of the gantry, as well as the LAO to RAO rotation, there is an automatic-stop safety feature of DARCA that can hinder its set-up and which sometimes requires the removal of intravenous tubing, sheets, and even arm boards. In the authors' experience, meticulous removal of the intravenous tubing and arm boards, if necessary before performing the safety sweep, can preclude this delay.

DARCA versus SA
DARCA thus represents a revolutionary advance in RA and is the latest huge leap forward for imaging science. Initial pilot studies have shown DARCA to be better both in terms of safety and a diagnostic capability when compared with SA.[29,30] Ongoing studies that should be available soon are needed to confirm the safety and efficacy of DARCA. In addition to safety studies, clearly the prolonged acquisition obtained during DARCA should permit, at least theoretically, the development of 3D-volumetric reconstruction. This is just one more

potential research application of this exciting technology that further highlights its potential.

SUMMARY

Catheter-based coronary angiography remains the diagnostic gold standard for CAD and represents one of the most common invasive procedures performed worldwide. Despite its widespread use, there are numerous limitations to standard static coronary angiography, which are related to its 2D luminology-like dataset, operator-dependent acquisitions, and the higher contrast volumes and radiations doses used to complete a study. RA was developed to overcome many of these known limitations. Technologic advancements, including the development of faster gantry rotations that are automated and flat-panel detectors, have permitted RA to become both clinically available and extremely efficacious. Numerous studies have been performed that have shown that RA indeed represents a leap forward in imaging science: that is, safer, faster, and angiographically better. Indeed, each study to date has shown a reduction in contrast use, which is critical given the aging population and the increasing prevalence of chronic kidney disease. There is also a decrease to neutral effect upon radiation exposure and procedural time with the use of RA, which further underscores its clinical safety and efficacy. In addition, RA has permitted numerous research advances, including modeling, gated- and motion-compensated, and automated 3D-volumetric reconstruction.

RA has continued to evolve, with its most recent development being dual-axis RA. This new technique further overcomes the numerous limitations of SA by providing additional views (**Fig. 5**). DARCA should be even better than single-axis RA by shortening LCA to just one acquisition. There are at least two ongoing studies of the clinical safety of this new type of RA, which should be available in 2009. Our current knowledge and expertise in all rotational modalities has allowed us to compare them to SA (**Table 1**).

The major hurdles for the widespread use of RA is the equipment upgrade and clinically focused training that is required for many contemporary laboratories, staff, and physicians, to be proficient in performing RA, as well as maximizing its clinical advantages. While RA is relatively inexpensive, the acquisition of new equipment can constitute a significant financial burden to many institutions with currently viable platforms. With the combination of several vendors offering rotational technology, numerous aging X-ray systems throughout the world, and emerging RA study results, it is anticipated that the next few years should show a greater penetrance of RA.

Overall, RA clearly provides numerous advantages over SA and has become the preferred method of coronary angiography at the authors' institution. With a very shallow learning curve,

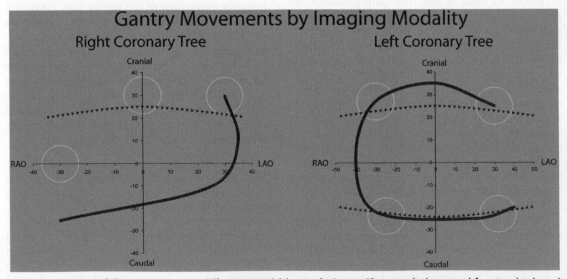

Fig. 5. Trajectories of the gantry arm in different acquisition techniques. The angulations used for standard angiography (SA) acquisitions are shown by red circles. The gantry trajectories based on single-axis rotational angiography (RA) is shown by the dotted lines. The solid line represents the continuous gantry angulations for dual-axis RA available on the X-per Swing Dual-axis RA product (Philips Health care, Best, The Netherlands).

Table 1
Comparison of different acquisition methods for coronary angiography

Angiography	Number of Acquisitions (LCA & RCA)	Total Number of Views	Contrast	Radiation	Time	3D Modeling Capability	3D Reconstruction Capability	Details
Standard Angiography	6–11	6–11	+	+	+	Yes	No	Multiple static projections
Single-axis rotational angiography	3	360° (120° per acquisition)	+++	+++	++/+++	Yes	No	Cranial and caudal rolls required for complete evaluation
180° rotational angiography	2	360° (180° per acquisition)	++	++	+	Yes	Yes	Single acquisition in PA projection
Dual-axis rotational angiography	2	Variable	+++	+++	++	Currently under investigation	Currently under investigation	Single acquisition of both cranial/caudal and LAO/RAO

This table displays each type of coronary angiography and its respective characteristics. All comparisons are made with respect to SA. Three-dimensional modeling is possible with all types of RA. Three-dimensional reconstruction with automated 3D capability is now possible with a 180° degree RA.
Abbreviations: +, Least favorable; ++, same; +++, most favorable. RAO = Right anterior oblique, LAO = left anterior oblique, 3-D = three dimensional, PA-posterior-anterior

operators can easily adapt these techniques, which have been shown to provide the optimal views of the coronary arteries while decreasing contrast use, radiation, and potentially procedural time.

APPENDIX: SUPPLEMENTARY MATERIAL

Supplementary material associated with this article can be found, in the on-line version, at doi:10.1016/j.ccl.2009.03.002.

REFERENCES

1. Green NE, Chen SY, Messenger JC, et al. Three-dimensional vascular angiography. Curr Probl Cardiol 2004;29(3):104–42.
2. Mintz GS, Painter JA, Pichard AD, et al. Atherosclerosis in angiographically "normal" coronary artery reference segments: an intravascular ultrasound study with clinical correlations. J Am Coll Cardiol 1995;25(7):1479–85.
3. Nissen SE, Gurley JC, Grines CL, et al. Intravascular ultrasound assessment of lumen size and wall morphology in normal subjects and patients with coronary artery disease. Circulation 1991;84(3):1087–99.
4. Ventura HO, White CJ, Jain SP, et al. Assessment of intracoronary morphology in cardiac transplant recipients by angioscopy and intravascular ultrasound. Am J Cardiol 1993;72(11):805–9.
5. Ramee SR, White CJ, Collins TJ, et al. Percutaneous angioscopy during coronary angioplasty using a steerable microangioscope. J Am Coll Cardiol 1991;17(1):100–5.
6. Teirstein PS, Schatz RA, DeNardo SJ, et al. Angioscopic versus angiographic detection of thrombus during coronary interventional procedures. Am J Cardiol 1995;75(16):1083–7.
7. Fearon WF, Takagi A, Jeremias A, et al. Use of fractional myocardial flow reserve to assess the functional significance of intermediate coronary stenoses. Am J Cardiol 2000;86(9):1013–4, A1010.
8. Pijls NH, De Bruyne B, Peels K, et al. Measurement of fractional flow reserve to assess the functional severity of coronary-artery stenoses. N Engl J Med 1996;334(26):1703–8.
9. White CW, Wright CB, Doty DB, et al. Does visual interpretation of the coronary arteriogram predict the physiologic importance of a coronary stenosis? N Engl J Med 1984;310(13):819–24.
10. Arnett EN, Isner JM, Redwood DR, et al. Coronary artery narrowing in coronary heart disease: comparison of cineangiographic and necropsy findings. Ann Intern Med 1979;91(3):350–6.
11. Schwartz JN, Kong Y, Hackel DB, et al. Comparison of angiographic and postmortem findings in patients with coronary artery disease. Am J Cardiol 1975;36(2):174–8.
12. Vlodaver Z, Frech R, Van Tassel RA, et al. Correlation of the antemortem coronary arteriogram and the postmortem specimen. Circulation 1973;47(1):162–9.
13. Green NE, Chen SY, Hansgen AR, et al. Angiographic views used for percutaneous coronary interventions: a three-dimensional analysis of physician-determined vs. computer-generated views. Catheter Cardiovasc Interv 2005;64(4):451–9.
14. Isner JM, Kishel J, Kent KM, et al. Accuracy of angiographic determination of left main coronary arterial narrowing. Angiographic–histologic correlative analysis in 28 patients. Circulation 1981;63(5):1056–64.
15. Topol EJ, Nissen SE. Our preoccupation with coronary luminology. The dissociation between clinical and angiographic findings in ischemic heart disease. Circulation 1995;92(8):2333–42.
16. Galbraith JE, Murphy ML, de Soyza N. Coronary angiogram interpretation. Interobserver variability. JAMA 1978;240(19):2053–6.
17. Scanlon PJ, Faxon DP, Audet AM, et al. ACC/AHA guidelines for coronary angiography. A report of the American College of Cardiology/American Heart Association Task Force on practice guidelines (Committee on Coronary Angiography). Developed in collaboration with the Society for Cardiac Angiography and Interventions. J Am Coll Cardiol 1999;33(6):1756–824.
18. Spears JR, Sandor T, Baim DS, et al. The minimum error in estimating coronary luminal cross-sectional area from cineangiographic diameter measurements. Cathet Cardiovasc Diagn 1983;9(2):119–28.
19. Tommasini G, Camerini A, Gatti A, et al. Panoramic coronary angiography. J Am Coll Cardiol 1998;31(4):871–7.
20. Maddux JT, Wink O, Messenger JC, et al. Randomized study of the safety and clinical utility of rotational angiography versus standard angiography in the diagnosis of coronary artery disease. Catheter Cardiovasc Interv 2004;62(2):167–74.
21. Akhtar M, Vakharia KT, Mishell J, et al. Randomized study of the safety and clinical utility of rotational vs. standard coronary angiography using a flat-panel detector. Catheter Cardiovasc Interv 2005;66(1):43–9.
22. Mehran R, Aymong ED, Nikolsky E, et al. A simple risk score for prediction of contrast-induced nephropathy after percutaneous coronary intervention: development and initial validation. J Am Coll Cardiol 2004;44(7):1393–9.
23. Kuon E, Niederst PN, Dahm JB. Usefulness of rotational spin for coronary angiography in patients

with advanced renal insufficiency. Am J Cardiol 2002;90(4):369–73.

24. Raman SV, Morford R, Neff M, et al. Rotational X-ray coronary angiography. Catheter Cardiovasc Interv 2004;63(2):201–7.

25. Garcia JA, Agostoni P, Green NE, et al. Rotational vs. standard coronary angiography: an image content analysis. Catheter Cardiovasc Interv 2009;73(6):753–61.

26. Rasche V, Movassaghi B, Grass M, et al. Automatic selection of the optimal cardiac phase for gated three-dimensional coronary x-ray angiography. Acad Radiol 2006;13(5):630–40.

27. Garcia JA, Chen SY, Messenger JC, et al. Initial clinical experience of selective coronary angiography using one prolonged injection and a 180 degrees rotational trajectory. Catheter Cardiovasc Interv 2007;70(2):190–6.

28. Garcia JA, Movassaghi B, Casserly IP, et al. Determination of optimal viewing regions for X-ray coronary angiography based on a quantitative analysis of 3D reconstructed models. Int J Cardiovasc Imaging 2008 [Epub ahead of print].

29. Klein AJ, Kim M, Casserly IP, et al. Safety and efficacy of XperSwing dual-axis rotational coronary angiography versus standard coronary angiography. Paper presented at: American College of Cardiology, Orlando, FL, 2009.

30. Horisaki T, Katoh O, Imai S, et al. Feasibility evaluation of dual axis rotational angiography (XperSwing) in the diagnosis of coronary artery disease. Medica-Mundi 2008;52(2):11–3.

Advances in Contrast Media and Contrast Injectors

John C. Messenger, MD*, Ivan P. Casserly, MB, BCh

KEYWORDS

- Contrast media • Contrast injectors
- Coronary angiography • Coronary imaging
- Contrast nephropathy

Although no contrast media approved by the Food and Drug Administration for coronary angiography have been introduced recently, several recent trials have assessed the safety of imaging agents in patients undergoing diagnostic and therapeutic iodinated contrast–based studies. Significant advances in coronary angiography have come through the introduction of techniques such as rotational angiography and the increasing use of automated contrast injectors in the catheterization laboratory. This article reviews the currently available agents used for contrast imaging during coronary angiography and intervention, recent data regarding potential adverse effects of contrast media, and ways to minimize the risks associated with their use. In addition, the authors review the state of the art in automated contrast injection for coronary angiography, including protocols used to perform rotational coronary angiography and digital subtraction imaging in the endovascular suite of the twenty-first century.

CONTRAST AGENTS
Background

The original contrast medium used for selective coronary angiography, introduced in the 1950s, consisted of sodium and meglumine salts of diatrizoic acid. The first agents were ionic and were classified as high osmolar contrast media (HOCM), with osmolality of five to eight times (> 1700 mOsm) that of blood. These contrast media had significant physiologic effects on both the hemodynamics and electrical activity of the heart and were associated with high rates of complications with selective injection into the coronaries including hypotension, arrhythmias, and volume overload. In the 1970s, low osmolar contrast media (LOCM, < 850 mOsm), became available with the modification of the benzoic acid side chain with an amide molecule, creating a non-ionic molecule. These molecules did not dissociate in solution, so there were three atoms of iodine for only one active particle, giving a ratio of 3:1 compared with ratios of 3:2 for HOCM. Adverse contrast reactions including nausea, vomiting, chest pain, and anaphylactoid reactions still were common with the initial LOCM agents. Not until the 1980s, with the advent of coronary intervention requiring significantly larger amounts of contrast, were newer contrast media developed that were considered safer and better tolerated by patients undergoing contrast-based studies.[1] At this time, a monoacid dimer was developed in which two tri-iodinated benzoic rings were linked together to create a non-ionic dimer. This linking resulted in six iodine atoms for the two active particles in each molecule, maintaining the same 3:1 ratio as in the monomers. In 1996, iodixanol, an iso-osmolar contrast medium (IOCM), was introduced. It is the only IOCM currently approved for use in the United States. The osmolality of iodixanol is similar to that of blood at an iodine concentration of 300 mg/mL, making it unique among contrast media used for angiography. The

Section of Interventional Cardiology, Division of Cardiology, University of Colorado Denver School of Medicine, 12401 E. 17th Avenue, Box B132, Aurora, CO 80045, USA
* Corresponding author.
E-mail address: john.messenger@ucdenver.edu (J.C. Messenger).

Cardiol Clin 27 (2009) 407–415
doi:10.1016/j.ccl.2009.03.003
0733-8651/09/$ – see front matter © 2009 Elsevier Inc. All rights reserved.

chemical structures discussed in this section are shown in **Fig. 1**.

Properties of Contrast Media Used for Coronary Angiography

Contrast media used for intravascular imaging have several important physiochemical properties related to ease of use, toxicity, and image quality. These characteristics include ionicity, osmolality, viscosity, and overall iodine content. Several of these characteristics have been implicated in the adverse reactions associated with the use of contrast media for coronary and peripheral vascular imaging. The route of administration of contrast medium is important, because these agents seem to be less nephrotoxic when given intravenously than when administered intra-arterially. The intrarenal concentration of contrast medium has been found to be much higher after an intra-arterial injection (with urinary concentrations 50 to 100 times that of circulating plasma levels) than after intravenous injection.[2] Because renal excretion is the major route of elimination for contrast media, the effects on renal function require attention: pre-existing renal insufficiency results in prolonged renal clearance of contrast, increasing the length of exposure to the chemotoxic properties of contrast media. The properties of these agents do seem to differ somewhat, even within classes of agents, and directly affect both renal function and the structural elements of the renal tubules.[3]

As a result of these reported differences, a myriad of clinical trials has assessed newer contrast agents in an attempt to determine the

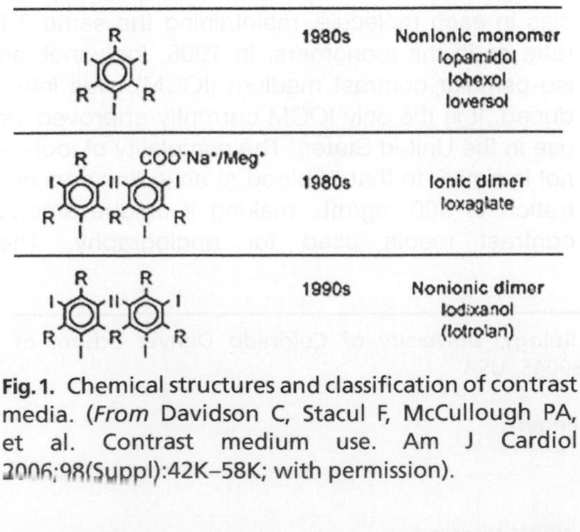

safest and most effective agent for intra-arterial applications. Given the many adverse events associated with the HOCM agents, most catheterization laboratories use either LOCM or IOCM for coronary angiography, because these agents are much better tolerated by patients, and their costs, which were prohibitively high originally, have decreased significantly. The properties of the most common contrast agents currently used for coronary angiography are shown in **Table 1**.

One of the challenges of introducing newer nonionic dimers has been an increase in viscosity that affects the ability to inject these agents effectively using standard manifold techniques. Although high viscosity is a feature of many contrast media at room temperature, the viscosity decreases markedly when the medium is warmed to 37°C, as is standard practice in most laboratories. The greater viscosity of some of the newer agents makes intravascular injection more difficult, particularly with hand injections through small catheters (4 French) for diagnostic angiography. This problem has been overcome to some degree by the introduction of automatic injector systems. As reported in the literature, the standard iodine concentrations used for coronary angiographic imaging are in the range of 270 to 350 mg iodine/mL and have not changed significantly during the last 20 years. With newer flat-panel detectors with improved image processing and enhancement software, however, contrast media with reduced iodine concentrations seem to have imaging characteristics comparable to those of contrast media with higher iodine concentrations. Studies are needed to see if reduced iodine concentration can reduce the incidence of adverse events related to the use of contrast media. The role of these properties (eg, ionicity, osmolality, iodine concentration) in adverse events remains quite controversial.

Adverse Events Associated with Contrast Media

Adverse reactions following the administration of contrast media related to the physicochemical properties outlined earlier have been classified as either idiosyncratic or chemotoxic.[4] Idiosyncratic reactions are anaphylactoid reactions that occur in an unpredictable fashion independent of the dose or the iodine concentration of the contrast media. The anaphylactoid nature of these reactions is thought to be secondary to the release of vasoactive mediators, including histamine. In general, the occurrence of these life-threatening reactions has decreased significantly with the introduction of LOCM and IOCM, occurring in

Molecular structure	Decade	Examples
COO⁻Na⁺/Meg⁺ CH₃CONH R	1950s	Ionic monomer Diatrizoate Iothalamate
R R R	1980s	Nonionic monomer Iopamidol Iohexol Ioversol
COO⁻Na⁺/Meg⁺ R R R	1980s	Ionic dimer Ioxaglate
R R R R	1990s	Nonionic dimer Iodixanol (Iotrolan)

Fig. 1. Chemical structures and classification of contrast media. (*From* Davidson C, Stacul F, McCullough PA, et al. Contrast medium use. Am J Cardiol 2006;98(Suppl):42K–58K; with permission).

Table 1
Characteristics of current contrast media

Name	Trade Name (Manufacturer)	Ionicity/Form	Type	Iodine Concentration (mg/mL)	Osmolality (mOsm/kg H₂O)	Viscosity at 37°C(mPa.s)
Iodixanol	Visipaque (GE Healthcare)	Non-ionic dimer	IOCM	320	290	11.8
Iomeprol[a]	Iomeron (Bracco International)	Non-ionic monomer	LOCM	350	620	7.5
Ioxaglate	Hexabrix (Covidien Imaging)	Ionic dimer	LOCM	350	680	10.5
Ioxilan	Oxilan (Guerbet)	Non-ionic monomer	LOCM	350	695	8.1
Iopamidol	Isovue (Bracco Diagnostics)	Non-ionic monomer	LOCM	350	730	7.0
Iopromide	Ultravist (Bayer Health care Pharmaceuticals)	Non-ionic monomer	LOCM	350	730	7.7
Iohexol	Omnipaque (GE Healthcare)	Non-ionic monomer	LOCM	350	780	10.6
Ioversol	Optiray (Covidien Imaging)	Non-ionic monomer	LOCM	350	790	8-9

Abbreviations: IOCM, iso-osmolar contrast medium; LOCM, low osmolar contrast medium.
[a] Not approved in the United States.

less than 0.05% to 0.1% of patients undergoing contrast-based imaging.[1] Chemotoxic reactions, on the other hand, are related to the dose, molecular structure, and physiochemical characteristics of contrast media. These reactions are more common and are dependent on many patient and procedure-related factors. The spectrum of these two types of reactions is shown in **Box 1**.

In general, predisposing factors for the development of anaphylactoid reactions include a history of prior contrast reaction, a history of asthma or bronchospasm, and general atopy. The presence of a seafood allergy is not related to an allergy to iodine but rather is associated with anaphylactoid reactions resulting from the atopic nature of the individual. Pretreatment of patients who have had prior contrast reactions with oral prednisone (40–60 mg orally) given 12 to 24 hours before the procedure and repeated along with oral diphenhydramine on the day of the procedure decreases the incidence of repeat reactions and should be incorporated into practice for patients who have risk factors for this potentially life-threatening event. Given the decreased frequency of these anaphylactoid reactions with newer contrast agents, it is important to understand the appropriate assessment and management, which Goss and colleagues[5] have reviewed for the Society of Cardiovascular Angiography and Interventions.

Chemotoxic events are quite common and include nausea, vomiting, pain during contrast injection, and decreased renal function. The most significant chemotoxic event associated with the use of contrast media is contrast-induced nephropathy (CIN), recently termed "contrast-induced acute kidney injury." The chemotoxic effects of contrast media are encountered most commonly in patients who have underlying renal impairment, diabetes mellitus, and markedly impaired cardiac function with decreased renal perfusion. A complete review of CIN is beyond the scope of this article, but the topic recently has been reviewed in depth.[6] One other important consideration when selecting a contrast medium is patient discomfort during injection, also a physiochemical effect thought to be related to osmolality. The pain experienced with IOCM versus LOCM agents has been studied; there is a decrease in perceived warmth and pain with the IOCM iodixanol.[7] Therefore iodixanol is the preferred contrast medium for ventriculography, aortography, internal mammary angiography, and for cerebral and peripheral angiography.

Contrast-induced nephropathy

CIN most commonly is defined as an increase in serum creatinine of 0.5 mg/dL or a 25% increase above the baseline value when assessed 48 hours after exposure to contrast medium. The incidence of CIN has decreased during the last decade, probably because of better risk assessment, improved contrast media with less renal toxicity, and attention to aggressive hydration and minimization of the dose of contrast medium. It is thought that the estimated glomerular filtration rate (eGFR) should be assessed in all patients undergoing coronary angiography and percutaneous coronary intervention (PCI), because the eGFR provides a much more accurate assessment of renal function than does the serum creatinine level.[6] CIN is most common in high-risk patients who have underlying chronic kidney disease (CKD), defined as an eGFR less than 60 mL/min/1.73 m^2.

The mechanism of renal injury in CIN is thought to result from decreased renal blood flow with stasis of contrast in the tubules allowing direct injury by the contrast medium. Unfortunately, many of the clinical trials examining CIN have been small and have been underpowered to detect a significant difference in outcomes. Multiple head-to-head studies have compared HOCM with LOCM, and recently the LOCM have been compared with IOCM. Given the small numbers in each study and the heterogeneity of the populations and procedures, the findings have been mixed.

Both the largest meta-analysis comparing HOCM and LOCM and the largest randomized trial in patients undergoing coronary angiography receiving either HOCM or LOCM showed a marked reduction (39% and 55%, respectively) in the development of CIN in patients receiving LOCM.[8,9] Importantly, the reduced rate of CIN seems to be limited to patients who have diabetes

---

Box 1
Types of reactions related to iodinated contrast media

Idiosyncratic
  Urticaria/hives
  Bronchospasm/wheezing
  Angioedema
  Laryngeal edema
  Hypotension/shock

Chemotoxic
  Nausea
  Vomiting
  Flushing
  Pain during injection
  Nephrotoxicity

mellitus and CKD or CKD alone. Diabetes alone, without the presence of pre-existing CKD, was not associated with increased risk of CIN in these studies.

Most studies assessing different LOCM agents have not demonstrated significant differences between these agents, probably because of small sample size.[10] The introduction of iodixanol in the mid-1990s resulted in multiple subsequent studies assessing its safety. Iodixanol is the only IOCM currently available in the United States. Several studies have shown it to have a lower risk of CIN than LOCM in patients who have CKD and diabetes mellitus undergoing coronary angiography.[11] This finding was confirmed by Solomon and colleagues,[12] who found the risk of CIN was lowest when iodixanol was used. Recently, however, the same investigators reported no difference in the risk of developing CIN in high-risk patients (eGFR 20–60 mL/min) undergoing coronary angiography receiving the IOCM iodixanol or the LOCM iopamidol.[13] Given the currently available evidence, the most recent guidelines for the management of acute coronary syndromes lists the use of IOCM as a class I recommendation (level of evidence A) for patients at risk for CIN.[14]

The development of CIN has important clinical effects because it increases the risk of both in-hospital and late mortality in patients receiving contrast media. The rates of CIN following diagnostic coronary angiography are difficult to determine, but CIN occurs almost exclusively in the presence of underlying renal impairment, particularly in the presence of diabetes mellitus. In patients undergoing PCI who have baseline renal impairment (serum creatinine ≥ 1.8 mg/dL) , the in-hospital mortality rate for patients who developed CIN was 14.9%, compared with 4.9% in patients who did not develop CIN. In addition, the development of CIN resulted in worsened outcomes following discharge, with a 1-year mortality of 37.7% in patients who had CIN versus 19.4% in those without CIN.[15] Multiple studies have shown that the volume of contrast medium, which is a modifiable factor, is an independent predictor of CIN. As a general rule, the contrast given during coronary angiography should not exceed two times the baseline eGFR.[16]

Strategies to reduce contrast nephropathy

Recently, the CIN Consensus Working Panel has published recommendations for decreasing the risk of CIN.[17] These recommendations include

1. The use of an iso-osmolar non-ionic contrast medium for angiography

2. Adequate volume expansion with isotonic crystalloid (0.9% normal saline) at 1 to 1.5 mL/kg/hour for 3 to12 hours before and 6 to 24 hours after exposure to contrast medium
3. Consideration of adjunctive agents (oral acetylcysteine, 600 mg–1200 mg twice daily, for two doses before and after contrast exposure ± sodium bicarbonate)

The role of adjunctive pharmacologic treatment is unclear at this time. Many early, small studies have demonstrated a reduction in rates of CIN, but several recent large trials of acetylcysteine and pre-hydration with sodium bicarbonate have demonstrated mixed results, with no clear benefit shown for these approaches compared with the use of aggressive hydration with normal saline in larger, randomized trials of coronary angiography.[18,19]

In patients who have CKD the amount of contrast medium should be limited to less than 30 mL for diagnostic studies and less than 100 mL for the diagnostic and PCI procedures. Reductions in the dose of contrast medium can be facilitated by changes in angiographic technique, including the use of rotational or biplane angiography and automated contrast injectors. Recently, a risk score for predicting of CIN following PCI has been developed and validated, allowing appropriate discussions with patients about the risks of developing CIN and the need for dialysis around the time of PCI.[20]

In an attempt to avoid further renal injury, there has been recent interest in using non-iodine–based imaging with the use of MRI agents such as gadolinium alone or gadolinium mixed with iodinated contrast medium for coronary angiography, because contrast media that do not contain iodine are thought to be less nephrotoxic. Multiple studies have demonstrated that diagnostic angiography can be performed satisfactorily with this strategy, although with less effective coronary opacification; this strategy, however, does not seem to decrease the incidence of CIN.[21]

Several interesting strategies that warrant further investigation involve the removal of the contrast medium following its use for coronary angiography and PCI. Recently, studies have assessed the impact of hemodialysis, hemofiltration, and novel contrast removal devices such as coronary sinus catheter systems that remove the contrast medium after it is delivered. All of these strategies are interesting means of reducing CIN, particularly in high-risk patients who have CKD, and have been reviewed recently in detail by McCullough.[6] Finally, as a parallel development, contrast media need to be improved further with reduced osmolality and less likelihood of chemotoxic adverse events.

Impact of Flat-Detector Technology on Coronary Imaging

In general, the image quality of coronary angiography has improved significantly with the introduction of digital imaging and the increasing penetrance of flat-detector technology. The contrast resolution, signal-to-noise ratio, and the dynamic range of imaging seems to be improved with flat-detector imaging, particularly with the advanced image processing software now available.[22]

With further improvements in software, it may be possible to improve imaging while using contrast media containing less iodine by using diluted contrast, by reducing osmolality and viscosity, or by using contrast media with lower iodine concentrations (150–270 mg/mL).

For example, one condition in which less dense coronary opacification may be important is during image acquisition with newer algorithms for three-dimensional volumetric reconstruction. These reconstructions are based on rotational angiographic acquisitions using flat-detector technology that require prolonged coronary injections (6–8 seconds) performed at reduced flow rates of 1.5 to 2.5 mL/sec, which can be performed easily and safely.[23,24] The impact of all these innovations on adverse events and image quality needs further investigation.

Integration of Contrast Injectors for Coronary Angiography

For the last 50 years, the standard for coronary angiography has been the stopcock-manifold system with hand injection of contrast using a syringe. Left ventriculography and aortography traditionally were performed by attachment to a power injector to inject a large-volume bolus. The initial injection systems used power injection with high volumes delivered at a fixed high-flow rate. Improved contrast injection systems have been introduced in the past decade that allow programmable, automated injection of contrast for coronary angiography (see **Fig. 2**).

The system that has been studied the most is the ACIST CVi (ACIST Medical Systems, Eden Prairie, Minnesota) injection system, which was introduced for coronary angiography as well as ventriculography and aortography. Now in its fourth generation, it provides programmable variable-rate contrast delivery with a hand-operated controller that allows a range of injection, from small puffs of contrast to large-volume bolus injections. It comes as a mobile or table-mounted single-injector system with a low profile.

Another system that has been introduced recently is the Avanta system (MEDRAD Inc., Warrendale, Pennsylvania), an automated fluid management system used for automated contrast injection in the catheterization laboratory. This system also is available as a table or pedestal-mounted system and features an injector system with separate contrast and saline tubing lines. These automated injection systems have built-in safety features including air-column detectors and pressure sensors to decrease the risk of barotrauma to the vessels injected.

Several recent studies have compared the safety and efficacy of these systems with standard manifold systems using hand injection. The programmable systems facilitate the use of smaller catheter size, particularly when 4-French systems are used with iso-osmolar contrast.[25] These systems have demonstrated equivalent images with significantly less contrast than used

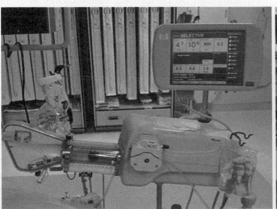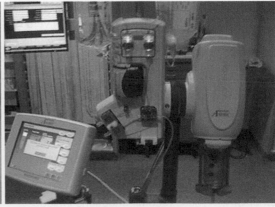

Fig. 2. Example of automated injectors used for coronary angiography. The CVi (ACIST Medical Systems, Eden Prairie, Minnesota) with touch-screen interface is shown in the left image. The Avanta (MEDRAD, Warrendale, Pennsylvania), also available as a table-side mount, is shown on the right.

Table 2
Proposed contrast delivery settings for automatic injectors

Imagine Modality	Vascular Bed	Flow Rates (mL/sec)	Total Volume (mL)	Pressure (PSI)	Rise Time
Static Imaging	LCA	3–4	8–10	500	0.5
	RCA	2–4	5–8	500	0.5
	LV	12–15	36–45	500–800	0.5–1
Rotational Imaging	LCA	2.5–4	10–16	500	0.5
	RCA	1.5–2.5	6–10	500	0.5
	LV	10–12	40–48	500–800	0.5–1
	SVG or IMA	2–3	8–12	500	0.5

Abbreviations: IMA, internal mammary artery; LCA, left coronary artery; LV, left ventriculography; RCA, right coronary artery; SVG, saphenous vein graft.

in standard techniques. Anne and colleagues[26] reported their experience in a randomized comparison of manual injection versus the use of the ACIST system for coronary angiography and PCI in 453 patients. There was a decrease in the total volume of contrast delivered to 49% of the patients undergoing coronary angiography and to 35% of the patients undergoing coronary angiography and PCI. Another recent study demonstrated a 25% reduction in contrast use and a 33% reduction in the rate of CIN after introduction of the ACIST system, compared with matched historical controls.[27]

These systems allow continuous hemodynamic monitoring during diagnostic and therapeutic procedures, except during injection, without the need for manifold and stopcock manipulation. The resulting "closed" system theoretically decreases the risk of air embolism caused by manifold malfunction or operator error. These systems also allow the operator to stand farther away from the imaging field, without leaning over the table or radiation source, thus reducing the operator's exposure to radiation.

These systems can deliver more compact boluses of contrast in a variable, controllable fashion that also serves to limit contrast-streaming artifacts. These systems also are necessary for rotational coronary and peripheral angiographic acquisitions, because they permit the prolonged, controlled, and synchronized injections needed for three-dimensional modeling and reconstruction. Through integrated interfaces, these systems also allow automated timing of injections with activation of the radiographic system. This synchronization is important for optimizing images for rotational coronary angiography and for digital subtraction angiography of the peripheral vasculature.

At this time, automated contrast management systems seem to have no disadvantages other than their initial cost. Overall, the published studies have shown cost savings with reduced contrast use and less waste than with traditional methods. There are minor differences between the currently available systems. For the catheterization laboratory staff, the set-up time is slightly longer initially than for standard manifold systems, but set-up speed increases with familiarity, especially with the built-in troubleshooting software available on the current systems. Integration into the catheterization laboratory is quite easy, with a relatively brief learning curve, and minimal troubleshooting is necessary once the staff is trained. The largest part of the learning curve involves the operator interaction with the tableside controls and optimizing injection protocols for patients. Injection settings must be individualized based on the size of the vascular structure being imaged (small versus large vessel, internal mammary artery, saphenous vein grafts, peripheral angiography). Some recommended injection parameters for coronary and peripheral angiography are outlined in **Table 2**. Overall, programmable, automated injection systems are important tools in the catheterization laboratory that help improve imaging, use less contrast medium, and allow operators to stay further from the x-ray source.

SUMMARY

Contrast media currently in use for coronary angiography and PCI are safer than prior generations, particularly with the introduction of LOCM and IOCM. With newer agents there has been a significant reduction in both anaphylactoid and chemotoxic adverse events. Despite the relative rarity of severe anaphylactoid reactions, understanding the prevention and emergent treatment of these potentially life-threatening events is critical.

Understanding the risk factors for the development of CIN and therapeutic strategies to minimize risks are important. The appropriate use of LOCM or IOCM in high-risk patients (eg, patients who have CKD, diabetes mellitus, or prior CIN) in conjunction with aggressive intravenous hydration, judicious use of contrast, and concomitant pharmacologic therapies can help minimize the risk of CIN. Future developments to minimize the risks of contrast media will focus on the development of less chemotoxic agents, with the goal of minimizing the risk of adverse events while optimizing imaging. Integration of automated contrast injector systems into the catheterization laboratory is associated with decreased contrast use, less contrast delivered to patients, and potentially a decreased risk of CIN as well. These systems have relatively brief learning curves and have the potential to decrease radiation exposure to the operators as well.

REFERENCES

1. Katayama H, Yamaguchi K, Kozuka T, et al. Adverse reactions to ionic and nonionic contrast media: a report from the Japanese Committee on the safety of contrast media. Radiology 1990;175:621–8.
2. Morcos SK, Thomsen HS, Webb JAW, et al. Contrast media induced nephrotoxicity: a consensus report. Eur Radiol 1999;9:1602–13.
3. Thomsen HS, Morcos SK. Radiographic contrast media. BJU Int 2000;86(suppl 1):1–10.
4. Pollack HM. History of iodinated contrast media. In: Thomsen HS, Muller RN, Mattrey RF, editors. Trends in contrast media. Berklin: Springer Verlag; 1999. p. 1–19.
5. Goss JE, Chambers CE, Heupler FA Jr. Systemic anaphylactoid reactions to iodinated contrast media during cardiac catheterization procedures: guidelines for prevention, diagnosis, and treatment. Laboratory Performance Standards Committee of the Society for Cardiac Angiography and Interventions. Cathet Cardiovasc Diagn 1995;34:99–104.
6. McCullough PA. Contrast-induced acute kidney injury. J Am Coll Cardiol 2008;51:1419–28.
7. Katayama H, Spinazzi A, Fouillet X, et al. Iomeprol: current and future profile of a radiocontrast agent. Invest Radiol 2001;36:87–96.
8. Barrett BJ, Carlisle EJ. Metaanalysis of the relative nephrotoxicity of high- and low-osmolality iodinated contrast media. Radiology 1993;188:171–8.
9. Rudnick MR, Goldfarb S, Wexler L, et al. Nephrotoxicity of ionic and non-ionic contrast media in 1196 patients: a randomized trial. Kidney Int 1995;47:254–61.
10. Davidson C, Stacul F, McCullough PA, et al. Contrast medium use. Am J Cardiol 2006;98:42K–58K.
11. Aspelin P, Aubry P, Fransson SG, et al. Nephrotoxic effects in high-risk patients undergoing angiography. N Engl J Med 2003;348:491–9.
12. Solomon R. The role of osmolality in the incidence of contrast-induced nephropathy: a systematic review of angiographic contrast media in high risk patients. Kidney Int 2005;68:2256–63.
13. Solomon RJ, Natarajan MK, Doucet S, et al. Cardiac Angiography in the Renally Impaired Patients (CARE) study: a randomized double-blind trial of contrast-induced nephropathy in patients with chronic kidney disease. Circulation 2007;115:3189–96.
14. Anderson JL, Adams CD, Antman EM, et al. ACC/AHA 2007 guidelines for management of patients with unstable angina/non-ST-elevation myocardial infarction—executive summary: a report of the American College of Cardiology/American Heart Association Task Force on practice guidelines (Writing Committee to Revise the 2002 Guidelines for Management of Patients with Unstable Angina/Non-ST-Elevation Myocardial Infarction). J Am Coll Cardiol 2007;50:652–726.
15. Gruberg L, Mintz GS, Mehran R, et al. The prognostic implications of further renal function deterioration within 48 h of interventional coronary procedures in patients with pre-existent chronic renal insufficiency. J Am Coll Cardiol 2000;36:1542–8.
16. Laskey WK, Jenkins C, Slezer F, et al. NHLBI dynamic registry investigators. Volume-to-creatinine ratio: a pharmacokinetically based risk factor for prediction of early creatinine increse after percutaneous coronary intervention. J Am Coll Cardiol 2007;50:584–90.
17. McCullough PA, Stacul F, Davidson C, et al. Overview. Am J Cardiol 2006;98:2K–4K.
18. Brar SS, Shen AY, Jorgensen MB, et al. Sodium bicarbonate vs sodium chloride for the prevention of contrast medium-induced nephropathy in patients undergoing coronary angiography: a randomized trial. JAMA 2008;300:1038–46.
19. Briguori C, Airoldi F, D'Andrea D, et al. Renal insufficiency following contrast media administration trial (REMEDIAL): a randomized comparison of 3 preventative strategies. Circulation 2007;115:1211–7.
20. Mehran R, Aymong ED, Nikolsky E, et al. A simple risk score for the prediction of contrast-induced nephropathy after percutaneous coronary intervention: development and initial validation. J Am Coll Cardiol 2004;44:1393–9.
21. Reed PS, Dixon SR, Boura JA, et al. Comparison of the usefulness of gadodiamide and iodine mixture versus iodinated contrast alone for prevention of

contrast-induced nephropathy in patients with chronic kidney disease undergoing coronary angiography. Am J Cardiol 2007;100:1090–3.

22. Holmes DR Jr, Laskey WK, Wondrow MA, et al. Flat-panel detectors in the cardiac catheterization laboratory: revolution or evolution—what are the issues? Catheter Cardiovasc Interv 2004;63:324–30.

23. Garcia JA, Chen SY, Messenger JC, et al. Initial clinical experience of selective coronary angiography using one prolonged injection and a 180 degrees rotational trajectory. Catheter Cardiovasc Interv 2007;70:190–6.

24. Hansis E, Schäfer D, Dössel O, et al. Projection-based motion compensation for gated coronary artery reconstruction from rotational x-ray angiograms. Phys Med Biol 2008;53:3807–20.

25. Chahoud G, Khoukaz S, El-Shafei A, et al. Randomized comparison of coronary angiography using 4F catheters: 4F manual versus "Acisted" power injection technique. Catheter Cardiovasc Interv 2001; 53:221–4.

26. Anne G, Gruberg L, Huber A, et al. Traditional versus automated injection contrast system in diagnostic and percutaneous coronary interventional procedures: comparison of the contrast volume delivered. J Invasive Cardiol 2004;16: 360–2.

27. Call J, Sacrinty M, Applegate R, et al. Automated contrast injection in contemporary practice during cardiac catheterization and PCI: effects on contrast-induced nephropathy. J Invasive Cardiol 2006;18:469–74.

Technique and Catheters

Ivan P. Casserly, MB, BCh[a],*, John C. Messenger, MD[b]

KEYWORDS

- Coronary angiography • Femoral access
- Radial access • Catheters • Coronary anomaly
- Native coronary artery • Coronary graft

Dramatic advances in the technique of coronary angiography have occurred since the first description by Sones and Shirey[1] in 1957. However, in 2009 the technique of coronary angiography and the range of catheters used to perform coronary angiography have reached a sufficient level of refinement such that current advances are generally of a minor nature. This article will review the current technique of coronary angiography focusing on the choice of arterial access site; navigation from the arterial access site to the ascending thoracic aorta; cannulation of the native coronary arteries in their normal, variant, and anomalous location; and cannulation of saphenous vein and arterial graft conduits.

ARTERIAL ACCESS
Which Access Site?

Worldwide, the vast majority of coronary angiographic procedures are performed using common femoral artery (CFA) access. However, in Europe and Asia, and to a lesser extent in the United States, an increasing percentage of cases are performed using radial artery access.[2] The relative advantages and disadvantages of each access are summarized in **Table 1**.

In general terms, radial artery access is technically more challenging, both in terms of placing a sheath in the smaller caliber radial artery, negotiating the path from the radial artery to the ascending aorta that may be influenced by anomalies in the anatomy of the upper extremity arteries and aortic arch, and cannulation of the coronary arteries.[2] Based on the experience of several centers and investigators, there is a longer learning curve for operators using radial access.[3,4] In addition, the ultimate success of programs seeking to institute a radial artery access program in the catheterization laboratory is predicated on a commitment to perform the majority of procedures using this route, and maintaining adequate operator volumes.[3,4]

The enthusiasm for radial artery access is driven by the desire to reduce significant CFA access site complications such as large groin hematoma, retroperitoneal hemorrhage, and pseudoaneurysm and arteriovenous fistula formation; and the data strongly supports this. A recent meta-analysis of randomized controlled trials comparing radial versus femoral access for coronary angiography and intervention demonstrated a 73% reduction in major bleeding associated with the use of radial access (0.05% versus 2.3%, OR 2.7, $P<.001$).[5] However, in a subgroup analysis of diagnostic-only studies, the major bleeding complication rate was equivalent in both groups, indicating that the major benefit of radial artery access is in the coronary intervention cohort.

Radial Artery Access—Technique

The patient's hand and forearm is placed on an arm board extending from the table, with the arm secured in a supine and slightly hyperextended position. A small amount (1–2 mL) of lidocaine is administered, and the radial artery is punctured approximately 1 to 2 m proximal to the styloid

[a] Department of Medicine, Division of Cardiology, University of Colorado Denver, Cardiac & Vascular Center–Mail Stop B-132, University of Colorado Hospital, Anschutz Medical Campus, Leprino Building, Room #524, 12401 E. 17th Ave., P.O. Box 6511, Aurora, CO 80045, USA
[b] Department of Medicine, Division of Cardiology, University of Colorado Denver, Cardiac & Vascular Center–Mail Stop B-132, University of Colorado Hospital, Anschutz Medical Campus, Leprino Building, Room #523, 12401 E. 17th Ave., P.O. Box 6511, Aurora, CO 80045, USA
* Corresponding author.
E-mail address: ivan.casserly@ucdenver.edu (I.P. Casserly).

Cardiol Clin 27 (2009) 417–432
doi:10.1016/j.ccl.2009.04.005

Table 1
Advantages and disadvantages of radial and femoral artery access for coronary angiography

	Radial Artery Access	Femoral Artery Access
Advantage	Reduced risk of bleeding complication Allows immediate ambulation Improved patient satisfaction and comfort Shortened hospital stay	Technically easier Higher procedural success

Disadvantage	Longer learning curve
	Radial access more technically challenging
	Coronary cannulation more difficult
	Procedural success reduced
	Possible increase in radiation exposure for
	  patient and operator
		Increased risk of bleeding and other access
		  site complications (eg, pseudoaneurysm
		  formation, arteriovenous fistula)
		More patient discomfort
		Delayed ambulation

process using a 21-gauss micropuncture needle (2.5 or 4 cm), through which a 0.018 in wire is advanced, allowing subsequent placement of an 8 to 10 cm sheath in the radial artery (**Fig. 1**). A variety of spasmolytic cocktails is used by different operators including nitroglycerin, verapamil, nicardipine, and papaverine to prevent radial artery spasm. Intravenous heparin is also administered directly into the arterial sheath to prevent thrombosis.

Common Femoral Artery Access—Technique

An important factor in minimizing the risk of arterial access complications from CFA access is the ability to achieve a single front wall arteriotomy in the CFA above the bifurcation. Using fluoroscopic localization of the femoral head as a landmark to guide the CFA puncture is an important component in this task (**Fig. 2**A). Studies have shown that the CFA bifurcation is superior to the middle of the femoral head in 99% of patients.[6] Hence, the optimal location for the CFA arteriotomy is a point above the middle of the femoral head and below the level of the inguinal ligament (see **Fig. 2**B). The body habitus of the patient will

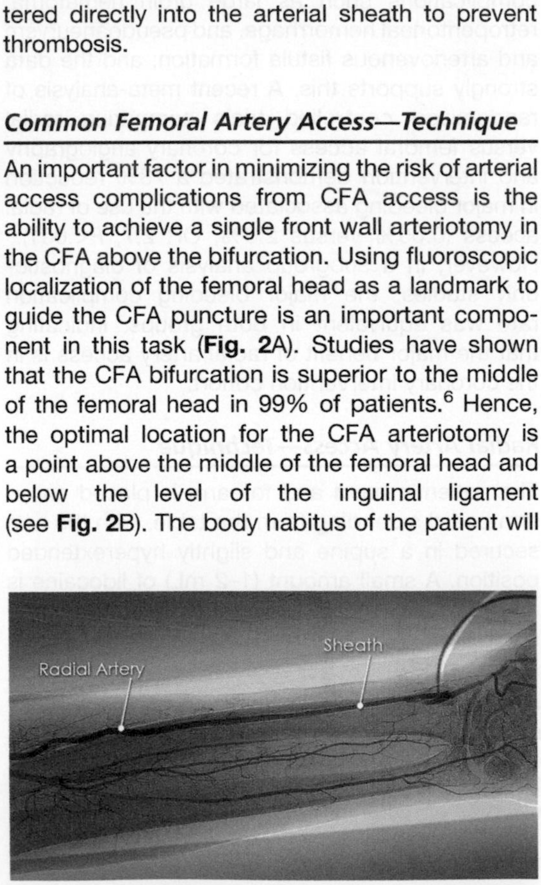

Fig. 1. Radial artery angiography following insertion of sheath in radial artery. Note the presence of spasm at the arteriotomy site.

significantly affect the horizontal distance between the skin puncture site and the arteriotomy site, with thinner patients having a short distance, and obese patients having a longer distance. When CFA access is performed without live fluoroscopic guidance, this distance needs to be taken into account even after fluoroscopic localization of the femoral head. In cases where the location of the arteriotomy is critical, live fluoroscopic guidance is recommended. Additionally, accurate digital localization of the CFA pulse and maximizing the transmitted pulsation from the needle tip before puncture is important in preventing side-wall or through-and-through sticks during access. In most laboratories, an 18-gauss needle (7–9 cm) is used to access the CFA, although a 21-gauss micropuncture system may also be used for patients with more challenging access.

Which Size Sheath?

The sheath size that is chosen is largely determined by the catheter size deemed necessary to achieve adequate opacification of the coronary artery or graft. With the miniaturization of catheter sizes, and the availability of automated injection systems that allow delivery of a fixed amount of contrast over a predefined time-period (see the article by Casserly and Messenger elsewhere in this issue for further exploration of this topic), good quality coronary angiography can be achieved in most patients using 4Fr sheaths.[7–9] For radial artery access, this is important because of the small caliber of some radial arteries; whereas, for femoral access, the decreased sheath size has a favorable impact on the bleeding risk and early ambulation. Situations in which larger catheter sizes and hence larger sheath sizes may be required include the presence of large caliber ectatic vessels, and high-output states (eg, aortic regurgitation).

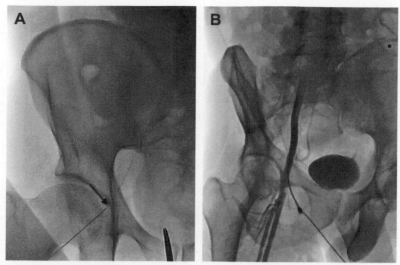

Fig. 2. Femoral artery access. (*A*) Fluoroscopic image showing an appropriate location of arterial puncture using the head of the femur as a landmark. The site of puncture of the CFA (*arrow*) with the micropuncture needle at a point just superior to the middle of the femoral head. (*B*) CFA angiography from a different patient following sheath insertion.

NAVIGATING FROM ARTERIAL ACCESS TO CORONARY OSTIUM
Common Femoral Artery Access

Navigating from the CFA to the ascending thoracic aorta is generally straightforward and achieved using 0.032 in to 0.038 in J-tipped wires supported by the appropriate diagnostic catheter. The most common challenges encountered include atherosclerotic aortoiliac disease, iliac tortuosity, and aortic aneurismal disease.

While occlusive disease of the aortoiliac territory precludes access, stenotic disease can often be negotiated by careful manipulation of wires and catheters. In general, a soft-tipped, 0.035 in wire, such as a Wholey, Magic Torque, or Rosen, supported by a Judkins right (JR) 4 or Bernstein catheter to allow steering of the wire, will negotiate the stenosis and allow catheter delivery. For the most severe stenoses, a 0.014 in interventional wire (eg, GrandSlam) may be required to cross the stenosis and angioplasty may be necessary to allow catheter delivery (**Fig. 3**). Knowledge of iliac anatomy is essential, and availability of radiograph equipment with digital subtraction capabilities and operators with expertise in peripheral angioplasty are very helpful in such situations.

Aortoiliac tortuosity is generally overcome by using soft-tipped, 0.035 in wires such as the Wholey, Magic Torque, or Rosen with a supporting catheter. However, in extreme situations, hydrophilic, 0.035 in glidewires with an angled tip may be required. The routine glidewire has a floppy body and is the safest first choice. Where more

support is required, an angled glidewire with a stiff body may be required.

Aortic aneurismal disease (generally infrarenal abdominal aneurysms) is not a contraindication to femoral access, but radial access should be considered for patients with the largest aneurysms, those with a history of thromboembolism, and those with evidence of severe angulation in the aneurysm. The strategy for negotiating these structures is to use soft-tipped, 0.035 in wires with a steerable supporting catheter (eg, JR 4 or Bernstein). Having crossed the aneurysm, a long femoral sheath (35–50 cm) should be placed such that the aneurysm is excluded from subsequent catheter exchanges, minimizing the risk of thromboembolism to visceral structures and the lower extremities.

Radial Artery Access

The challenges faced during navigation from the radial artery access site to the ascending thoracic aorta are distinct from those encountered using CFA access. Anatomic variations of the upper limb arteries are common, occurring in 10% to 20% of patients, and include the presence of radial stenosis or hypoplasia, radial artery loops, abnormal origin of the radial artery (most commonly from the brachial artery, **Fig. 4**A), severe tortuosity of the subclavian or innominate artery, and anomalous origin of the right subclavian artery from the aortic arch (lusoria subclavian artery, **Fig. 4**B).[10–13] These variations

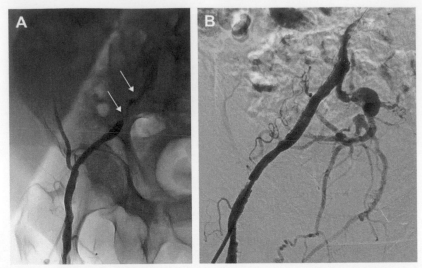

Fig. 3. (*A*) Severe external iliac artery disease (*arrows*) in a patient with attempted right CFA access. (*B*) External iliac artery angiography following angioplasty and stent placement, allow subsequent CFA access and performance of coronary angiography.

underlie the increased technical challenge and the longer learning curve associated with radial access.

Achieving success in the face of these anatomic variations is predicated on awareness, and prompt detection by using angiography (preferably digital subtraction) when any difficulty with wire or catheter advancement is encountered. Some operators perform routine angiography before any attempt to deliver wires or catheters. A complete description of the techniques used to overcome all of these anatomic variations is beyond the scope of this article. In general, negotiation of radial tortuosity and radial loops requires the use

of 0.014 in coronary hydrophilic wires (eg, Choice PT, Whisper), whereas 0.035 in hydrophilic glide-wires are required to negotiate tortuosity in the larger caliber axillary and innominate arteries. The use of hydrophilic catheters may also facilitate catheter delivery over these wires in this circumstance. Radial artery stenosis or hypoplasia may preclude catheter delivery depending on the severity and extent of luminal narrowing. Angioplasty of a focal radial artery stenosis may be reasonable in some circumstances to allow catheter delivery. Overcoming the acute angulation associated with an anomalous origin of the right subclavian artery from the aortic arch may require

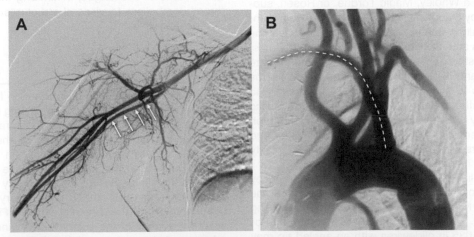

Fig. 4. Anomalies of upper extremity arterial anatomy. (*A*) Anomalous origin of the radial artery from the proximal brachial artery (*arrows*). (*B*) Anomalous origin of the right subclavian artery from the aortic arch distal to the origin of the left subclavian artery (*dotted line*).

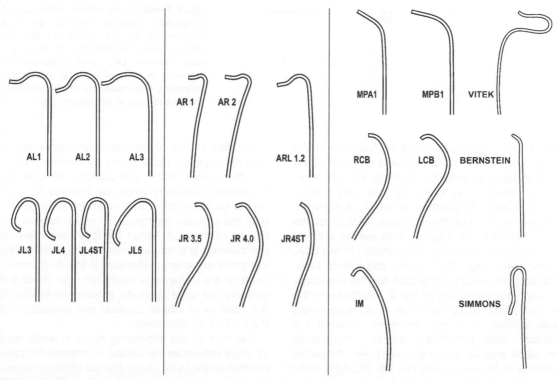

Fig. 5. Diagnostic catheters used to perform angiography of native coronary arteries and coronary grafts. AL, Amplatz left; AR, Amplatz right; IM, internal mammary; JL, Judkins left; JR, Judkins right; LCB, left coronary bypass; MPA, multipurpose A; MPB, multipurpose B; RCB, right coronary bypass; ST, short tip.

several maneuvers to achieve successful catheter delivery to the ascending aorta.

CANNULATION OF NATIVE CORONARY ARTERIES

Cannulation of the right and left coronary arteries is performed using a variety of catheters with distinct preformed shapes (**Fig. 5**). For the vast majority of catheters, the shape difference refers to variation in a single plane. A small number of catheters have variation in shape in a third dimension. These are typically used for the most difficult cannulations. In describing the shape of catheters, a common terminology is employed. The primary curve refers to the curve closest to the catheter tip, whereas secondary and tertiary curves refer to subsequent curves along the length of the catheter (**Fig. 6**). The goal of cannulation is to align the tip of the catheter in a coaxial fashion with the origin of the coronary artery, and record a normal continuous arterial pressure waveform from the catheter tip before injection of contrast for vessel opacification (**Fig. 7**). Understanding the variety of catheter types available, learning how to manipulate these catheters, and adapting the catheter choice to the individual anatomy of each patient are essential elements in achieving high success rates for coronary cannulation with minimal

complications (**Table 2**). In addition, where a diagnostic catheter will not successfully engage a coronary artery ostium, the authors will use a guide catheter with the desired shape.

Left Coronary Artery

The ostium of the left coronary artery (LCA) generally arises from the middle portion of the left coronary sinus, just inferior to the sinotubular junction, and the proximal segment of the artery pursues an orthogonal course with respect to the sinus (**Fig. 8**).[14] In such situations, a Judkins left (JL) 4 catheter will successfully engage this ostium with

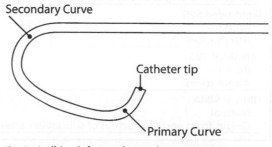

Fig. 6. Judkins left 4 catheter demonstrating nomenclature of the primary and secondary curves.

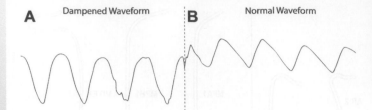

A Dampened Waveform   B   Normal Waveform

Fig. 7. Pressure waveform from tip of diagnostic catheter, initially showing dampening of the waveform due to lack of coaxial alignment with the coronary ostium (*A*), and subsequently showing a normal arterial waveform following manipulation of the catheter to achieve coaxial alignment (*B*).

little or no manipulation (**Fig. 9**). Variation in the origin and course of the proximal segment of the LCA in both an anterior-posterior and superior-inferior direction is common, and may require some subtle manipulation of the JL 4 catheter. Clockwise and counterclockwise rotation of the JL 4 catheter will typically address an anterior and posterior location and orientation of the LCA, respectively (**Fig. 10**). Superior and inferior location and orientation of the LCA may be overcome through manipulations of the JL 4 catheter in the vertical plane, or by the use of JL curve catheters with smaller or larger distances between the primary and secondary curves, respectively (ie, JL 3 and JL 5, respectively). An alternative strategy is to use an Amplatz left (AL)-type catheter (**Fig. 11**). This catheter is delivered to the

aortic root such that the secondary curve of the catheter typically rests in the noncoronary sinus and the primary curve and catheter tip is in the left anterior coronary sinus. By pushing forward on the catheter with some counterclockwise torque, the catheter tip moves superiorly toward the ostium of the LCA. When the final movement of the catheter is a forward motion, the catheter tip will point superiorly; whereas, if the final movement of the catheter is backward, the tip of the catheter will point inferiorly, allowing variations in the superior or inferior location and orientation of the LCA to be overcome.

The size of the ascending thoracic aorta also strongly influences the choice of catheter for cannulation of the LCA. Under normal circumstances, the secondary curve of the JL catheter rests

Table 2
Summary of catheter types used to engage native coronary arteries and grafts during coronary angiography

Coronary Artery or Graft	Catheter Type
RCA	
Normal origin and course	JR 4
Anterior ectopic origin	AR, Hockey stick, AL
Inferior ectopic origin with inferior course	Multipurpose
Superior ectopic origin from ascending thoracic aorta with inferior course	Multipurpose
Superior course	IM, superior right
Anomalous RCA from left sinus	JL 5,6, AR 2,3, Leya
LCA	
Normal origin and course	JL 4
Large ascending thoracic aorta	JL 5, JL 6
Small ascending thoracic aorta	JL 3
Anomalous origin from right sinus	AR
Anomalous origin of LCx from right sinus	JR, AR, multipurpose
Right-sided SVG	
Routine	Multipurpose
Alternatives	JR, right coronary bypass, AR
Left-sided SVG	
Routine	JR
Alternatives	left coronary bypass, AL
LIMA or RIMA	
Normal	IM
Origin from vertical portion of subclavian artery	JR 4, Bernstein

Abbreviations: AL, Amplatz left; AR, Amplatz right; IM, internal mammary; LCx, left circumflex; LIMA, left internal mammary; RCA, right coronary artery; RIMA, right internal mammary.

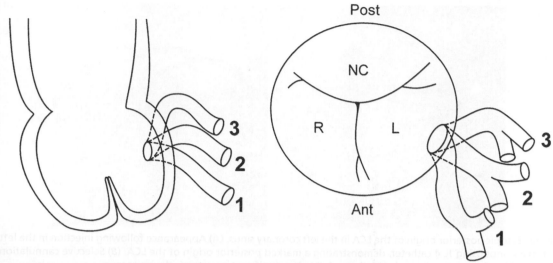

Fig. 8. Schematic demonstrating the typical origin of the LCA from the left coronary sinus and some variations in the course of the proximal segment. Ant, anterior; L, left; NC, non-coronary; Post, posterior; R, right.

against the midportion of the contralateral wall of the ascending thoracic aorta (see **Fig. 9**). In patients with a very large aorta (eg, ascending thoracic aortic aneurysm), the contact point of the secondary curve moves inferiorly toward the coronary sinus, resulting in a vertical orientation of the catheter tip (**Fig. 12**), which can result in

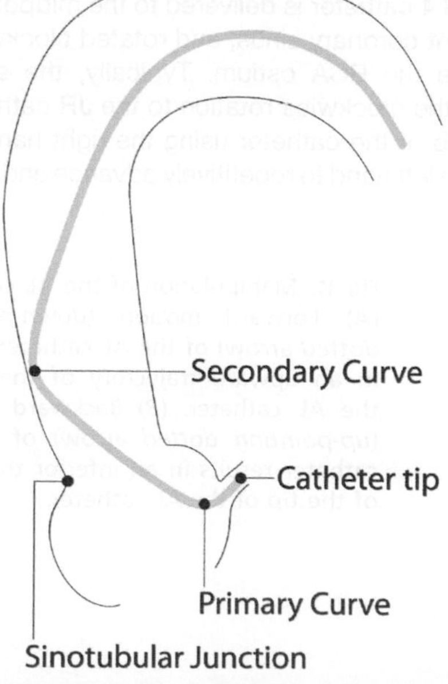

failure of the catheter tip to be coaxial with the LCA ostium, increasing the likelihood of coronary dissection if injections are performed with the catheter in this position. The solution to this problem is to use a JL catheter with a larger distance between the primary and secondary curve (see **Fig. 12**). Similarly, for patients with small diameters of the ascending thoracic aorta, the secondary curve of the JL 4 catheter will contact the aorta near the horizontal portion of the arch resulting in a very horizontal or inferior orientation of the catheter tip that can make cannulation of the LCA difficult (**Fig. 13**). The solution to this problem is to use a JL catheter with a shorter distance between the primary and secondary curves (see **Fig. 13C**).

Anomalies of the native coronary arteries refer to variations that occur with a frequency of less than 1%.[14] Separate ostia of the left anterior descending and left circumflex arteries are seen in approximately 0.7% of individuals. The left anterior descending (LAD) ostium will generally be engaged using a JL-type catheter with a shorter distance between the primary and secondary curve (ie, JL 3), with clockwise movement of the tip, whereas the left circumflex (LCx) ostium is often engaged using a JL-type catheter with a longer distance between the primary and secondary curve (ie, JL 5), with counterclockwise movement of the tip (**Fig. 14**). Similar strategies can be employed when faced with a patient with a very short left main coronary artery, where selective engagement of the LAD and LCx arteries is often required to opacify each vessel.

Secondary Curve

Catheter tip

Primary Curve

Sinotubular Junction

Fig. 9. Schematic of the aortic arch in the left anterior oblique projection showing the normal position of the JL 4 catheter in a patient with normal size of the ascending thoracic aorta and normal origin of the LCA.

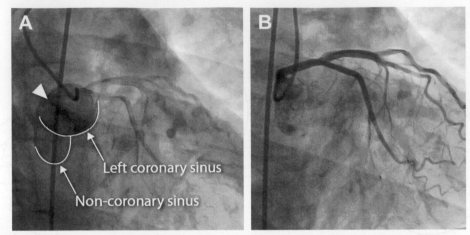

Fig. 10. Ectopic posterior origin of the LCA in the left coronary sinus. (*A*) Appearance following injection in the left coronary sinus using JL 4 catheter, demonstrating a marked posterior origin of the LCA. (*B*) Selective cannulation of the LCA using an Amplatz left 2 catheter following significant counterclockwise torque.

The circumflex artery may arise from the right coronary sinus or the proximal portion of the right coronary artery (RCA). This anomaly occurs with a frequency of approximately 0.7%. Typically, the proximal portion of such an anomalous vessel has an inferior course. Based on case series of diagnostic angiography and interventions in such patients, a variety of catheter types including JR, Amplatz right (AR), and multipurpose may be used to selectively engage an anomalous LCx arising from the right coronary sinus (**Figs. 15** and **16**).[15] Finally, the LCA may arise entirely from the right coronary sinus. This is the least common anomaly of the LCA, occurring in approximately 0.15% of individuals. Rare case reports of interventions in such anomalous vessels suggest that AR catheter types will successfully engage this vessel.[16]

Right Coronary Artery

The ostium of the RCA generally arises from the middle portion of the right coronary sinus, just inferior to the sinotubular junction, and the proximal segment of the artery generally pursues an orthogonal course with respect to the sinus (**Fig. 17**). A JR 4 catheter will successfully engage the RCA ostium in most patients. However, in contrast to the engagement of the LCA ostium with the JL 4 catheter, engagement of the RCA ostium with the JR 4 catheter requires significantly more manipulation. The JR 4 catheter is delivered to the midportion of the right coronary sinus, and rotated clockwise to engage the RCA ostium. Typically, the authors apply the clockwise rotation to the JR catheter at the hub of the catheter using the right hand, and use the left hand to repetitively advance and retract

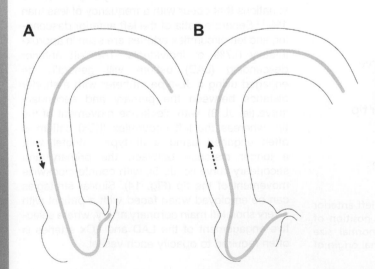

Fig. 11. Manipulation of the AL catheter. (*A*) Forward motion (*down-pointing dotted arrow*) of the AL catheter results in an upward trajectory of the tip of the AL catheter. (*B*) Backward motion (*up-pointing dotted arrow*) of the AL catheter results in an inferior trajectory of the tip of the AL catheter.

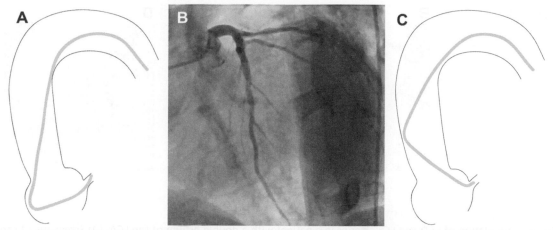

Fig. 12. Cannulation of the LCA in patients with large ascending thoracic aorta. (*A*) Schematic of the typical behavior of a JL 4 catheter in a patient with a large ascending thoracic aorta, with the secondary curve in the contralateral coronary sinus and the tip of the catheter assuming a vertical trajectory in the roof of the LCA. (*B*) Angiogram illustrating the vertical trajectory of a JL 4 catheter tip in a patient with a large ascending thoracic aorta. (*C*) Schematic of the behavior of a JL catheter with a larger distance between the primary and secondary curves.

the JR catheter over short distances to facilitate transmission of the torque to the catheter tip.

Variations in the location of the RCA ostium and orientation of the proximal segment are common (**Fig. 18**). The most common variations in location include an anterior, low ectopic, or high ectopic origin of the RCA ostium. Catheters with a longer reach than the JR 4 are often required to engage the RCA with an anterior origin (see **Fig. 18**), and include AR, AL, and hockey stick catheters. A multipurpose catheter is often successful for engagement of the RCA with its ostium located low in the

right coronary sinus with a horizontally directed proximal segment, or a high ectopic origin from the ascending aorta with an inferiorly directed proximal segment. For superiorly oriented RCA origins (ie, shepherd's crook), an internal mammary (IM), superior right, or AR catheter may be used.

Anomalous origin of the RCA from the left coronary sinus (ARCA) occurs in approximately 0.9% of individuals undergoing coronary angiography. Typically, the ostium of this artery lies anterior and superior to the origin of the LCA, and the proximal segment has an abrupt downward and

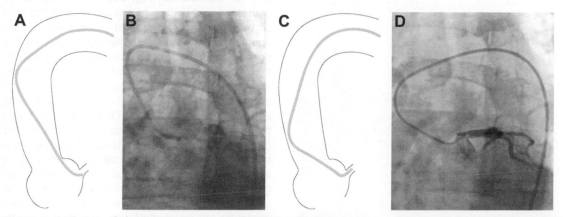

Fig. 13. Cannulation of the LCA in patients with small ascending thoracic aorta. (*A*) Schematic of the typical behavior of a JL 4 catheter in a patient with a small ascending thoracic aorta, with the secondary curve resting high in the ascending aorta near the horizontal portion of the arch and the tip of the catheter assuming a horizontal trajectory at the ostium of the LCA. (*B*) Angiogram illustrating the horizontal trajectory of a JL 4 catheter tip in a patient with a small ascending thoracic aorta. (*C*) Schematic of the behavior of a JL catheter with a shorter distance between the primary and secondary curves. (*D*) Angiogram illustrating the coaxial trajectory of a JL 3 catheter tip in a patient with a small ascending thoracic aorta.

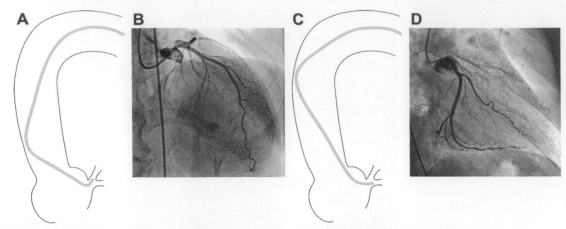

Fig. 14. Cannulation of LAD and LCx arteries in a patient with a double ostium of the LCA. (*A*) Schematic of cannulation of the LAD ostium using a JL catheter with a shorter distance between the primary and secondary curve. (*B*) Selective angiography of the LAD. (*C*) Schematic of cannulation of the LCx ostium using a JL catheter with a longer distance between the primary and secondary curve. (*D*) Selective angiography of the LCx.

rightward course as the vessel passes between the aorta and pulmonary artery toward the right atrioventricular groove. The latter anatomic feature can result in a slit-like orifice of this vessel, which can compound the technical challenge of engaging the ostium. Based on the authors' experience, and extrapolating from a number of case reports that describe the guide catheter type used to perform interventions to treat disease in ARCAs, the catheters that are typically successful in engaging ARCA include JL 4, 5, and 6, and AL 2 and 3 (**Fig. 19**).[17,18] A novel group of diagnostic catheters and interventional guides have been developed by Leya and colleagues[19] that are

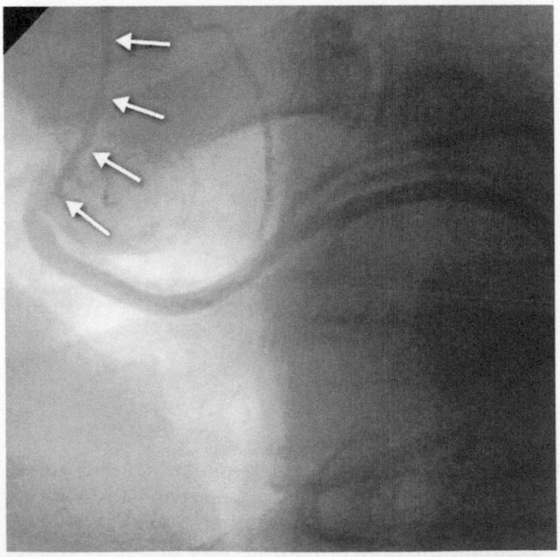

designed specifically to cannulate ARCA. These catheters have an AL or modified Judkins shape, with a tip that is directed both anterior and to the right at either 45° or 90°. The clinical experience of this group with these novel catheter and guides supports their utility for this difficult anomaly.[19]

CANNULATION OF GRAFTS
Right-Sided Vein Grafts

Right-sided vein grafts are typically sewn to the right side of the ascending thoracic aorta and the proximal segment has an inferior course. As a result, the authors' preference is to attempt engagement of these grafts in the left anterior oblique projection, and to use a multipurpose catheter for cannulation (**Fig. 20**). The multipurpose catheter is advanced to the ascending thoracic aorta to the anticipated level of the graft, rotated counterclockwise until the tip points toward the right side of the aorta. Maintaining this orientation, the catheter is then moved superiorly and inferiorly along the length of the right side of the aorta with slight variation in rotation of the catheter if the initial attempts are unsuccessful. Other catheters types that may be employed include JR 4, AR, and right coronary bypass. The importance of coaxial alignment of the catheter tip with the graft is critical, as in the authors' experience, some right-sided vein grafts are labeled as being occluded or as having severe ostial disease when catheters with a horizontal tip are malaligned with a marked inferiorly directed proximal segment (see **Fig. 20**C).

Left-Sided Vein Grafts

Left-sided vein grafts are typically sewn to the anterior wall of the ascending thoracic aorta and

Fig. 15. Anomalous origin of the LCA from the right coronary sinus. Arrows indicate the position of the multipurpose catheter used to cannulate this vessel.

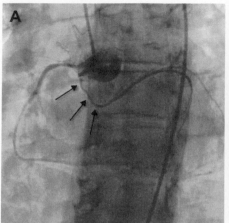 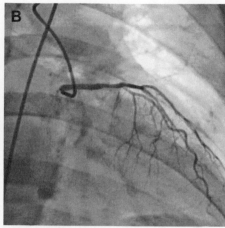

Fig. 16. (*A*) Angiography using JR 4 catheter with selective engagement of anomalous LCx artery (*arrows*). (*B*) Angiography of the LCA, demonstrating typical appearance of apparent long, left main coronary artery (actually the LAD because of the anomalous origin of the LCx artery). Note the posterior ectopic origin of the LAD in the left coronary sinus in this right anterior oblique view.

the proximal segment has a superior or horizontal course. As a result, the authors' preference is to engage these grafts in the right anterior oblique (RAO) projection (**Fig. 21**). An initial attempt to engage the graft with a JR 4 catheter is made. If unsuccessful, an understanding of the mechanism of failure is sought by injecting contrast though the catheter in the aorta. The two most common reasons for failure with the JR 4 catheter is an inability to reach the anterior wall of the aorta and failure of the horizontal orientation of the JR catheter tip to align with a superiorly oriented graft. If either of these anatomic features is seen, then a left coronary bypass catheter will typically be successful. AL catheters are also very useful for superiorly oriented left-sided grafts, and for engaging left-sided grafts that have been sewn high on the ascending thoracic aorta (usually because of heavy calcification in the lower ascending thoracic aorta).

Internal Mammary Artery Grafts

The left IM artery (LIMA) arises as the second branch from the first segment of the subclavian artery. In most patients, the ostium of the LIMA is located in the horizontal portion of the subclavian artery, just distal to where the vessel changes from a vertical toward a horizontal course, and has an anterior and inferior location at that point.

Selective engagement of the left subclavian artery is a necessary prerequisite to selective LIMA angiography. In most patients, this is achieved using a JR 4 catheter, by applying counterclockwise torque while withdrawing the catheter from the horizontal portion of the aortic arch.

Alternatively, a Bernstein catheter, which has a short tip with less acute angulation compared with a JR 4 catheter, may be used (see **Fig. 5**). In patients with more difficult arch anatomies (eg, Type III aortic arch), a Vitek or Simmons catheter

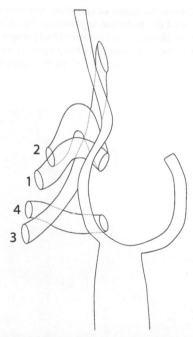

Fig. 17. Typical origin of the RCA from the right coronary sinus and some variations in both the location and the course of the proximal segment. (1) normal anatomic origin and course of the RCA, (2) superior course of proximal segment of RCA (Shepherd's Crook), (3) ectopic origin of RCA superior to sinotubular junction, (4) low ectopic origin of RCA.

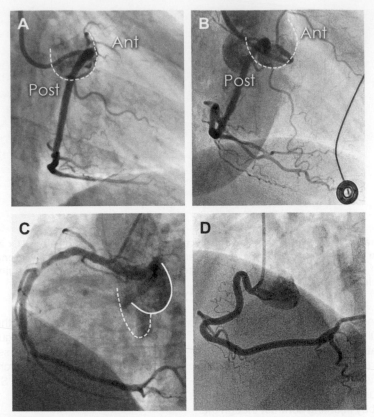

Fig. 18. Clinical examples of variation in the location of the ostium of the RCA within the right coronary sinus and the course of the proximal segment of the RCA. (*A*) Anterior (Ant) origin of the RCA with successful cannulation using an AR catheter. (*B*) Posterior (Post) origin of the RCA. (*C*) Superior ectopic origin above the sinotubular junction. (*D*) Superior course (shepherd's crook) of the proximal segment of the RCA. Right coronary sinus indicated by dotted lines. Left coronary sinus indicated by solid line.

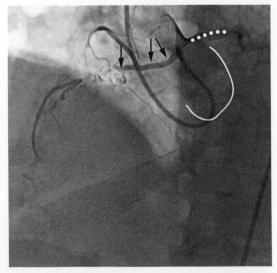

Fig. 19. Anomalous origin of the RCA from the left coronary sinus (*black arrows*). Left coronary sinus (*solid line*), and course of left main coronary artery (*dotted line*).

may be required (see **Fig. 5**). Selective angiography of the left subclavian artery is recommended before an attempt at LIMA angiography for two primary reasons: it allows an assessment for the presence of subclavian artery stenosis, and it demonstrates the anatomic features of the left subclavian artery and LIMA origin that may influence the technique used to achieve selective engagement of the LIMA (**Fig. 22**).

Following engagement and angiography of the left subclavian artery, a 0.035 in J-tipped wire is typically advanced to the axillary artery, allowing delivery of the diagnostic catheter to the second or third segment of the subclavian artery. Severe tortuosity of the left subclavian artery may require the use of a soft-tipped wire (eg, Wholey, Rosen, Magic Torque) or a glidewire to negotiate the tortuosity. The JR 4 catheter is then exchanged for an IM catheter, whose inferiorly directed tip is more suited to cannulation of the LIMA ostium. With the image intensifier in the RAO projection (since this displays the LIMA ostium optimally), the IM catheter is withdrawn slowly and when the

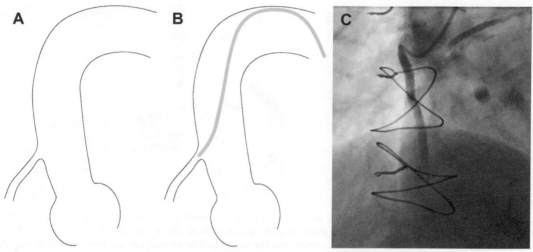

Fig. 20. Cannulation of right-sided saphenous vein grafts (SVG). (*A*) The aortic arch in the LAO projection showing the typical origin of the right-sided SVG from the right side of the ascending thoracic aorta with an inferior course of the proximal segment. (*B*) Coaxial cannulation of the right-sided SVG with a multipurpose catheter. (*C*) Angiogram showing lack of coaxial alignment of the horizontal tip of the JR 4 catheter with the origin of a right-sided SVG.

catheter tip nears the apparent location of the LIMA ostium, the IM catheter is rotated counter-clockwise to move the tip in an anterior direction.

When a Vitek or Simmons catheter is required to engage the left subclavian artery, these catheters may need to be exchanged for a Bernstein or JR 4 after delivery of the 0.035 in wire to the axillary artery because the inherent shape of these catheters make catheter delivery difficult and

sometimes impossible. In situations where the LIMA has an origin from the vertical portion of the subclavian artery, a diagnostic catheter with a more horizontal tip compared with the IM catheter (eg, JR 4, Bernstein) may be more successful.

The anatomy of the right IM artery (RIMA) is similar to that described for the LIMA, except that the right subclavian artery arises from the innominate artery rather than directly from the aortic

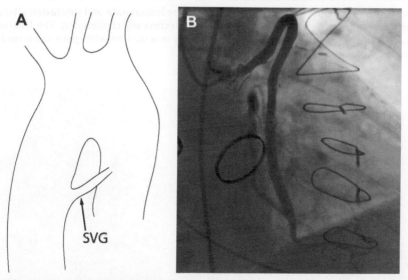

Fig. 21. Cannulation of left-sided saphenous vein grafts (SVG). (*A*) The aortic arch in the RAO projection showing the typical origin of the left-sided SVG from the anterior wall of the ascending thoracic aorta with an superior course of the proximal segment. (*B*) Coaxial cannulation of the left-sided SVG with a left coronary bypass catheter.

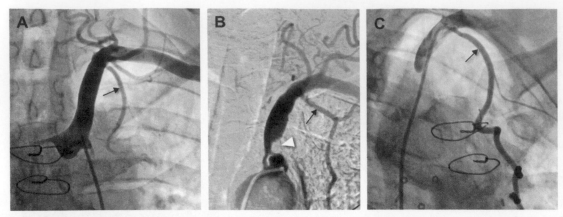

Fig. 22. LIMA angiography. (*A*) Nonselective angiogram of the left subclavian artery demonstrating absence of disease in the left subclavian artery and location of LIMA (*black arrow*). (*B*) Nonselective angiogram of the left subclavian artery showing eccentric severe stenosis near the origin (*white arrow*). Location of LIMA (*black arrow*). (*C*) Selective angiogram of LIMA (*black arrow*) shown in (*A*) using IM catheter.

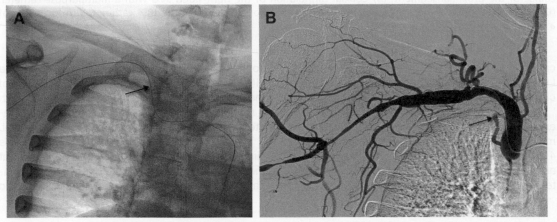

Fig. 23. RIMA angiography. (*A*) Note the marked tortuosity in the innominate and subclavian artery demonstrated by the course of the wire, making cannulation of the RIMA technically challenging. The location of the RIMA ostium shown by the arrow. (*B*) Subclavian artery angiography in a patient with giant-cell arteritis. The location of the RIMA shown by the arrow.

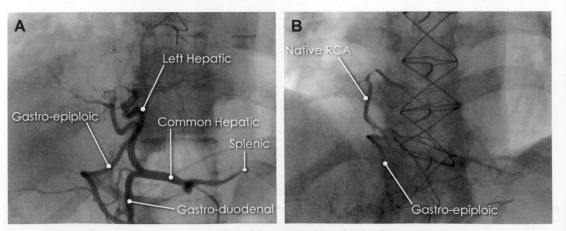

Fig. 24. Angiography of the gastroepiploic artery. (*A*) Angiography of the inflow to the gastroepiploic artery. (*B*) Angiography of the gastroepiploic artery and its distal target in the RCA.

arch. As a result, although the technical considerations are similar to those just described for cannulation of the LIMA, the technique for cannulation of the RIMA is more challenging (**Fig. 23**). In a patient who is known to have a RIMA graft, it is important to determine before angiography whether the RIMA was left in situ, or was taken down and sewn to the ascending thoracic aorta, where it will typically be attached to the anterior wall of the aorta and be used to bypass a branch of the LCA.

GASTROEPIPLOIC ARTERY GRAFT ANGIOGRAPHY

The gastroepiploic artery is typically grafted onto a vessel on the inferior wall of the heart, and is used in situations where other grafts are not available or have been exhausted in prior coronary bypass surgeries. Cannulation of this graft requires an understanding of the anatomy of the celiac trunk and some experience with cannulating the mesenteric arteries (**Fig. 24**).

An initial aortogram in the lateral projection to identify the location of the celiac trunk and assess for the presence of atherosclerotic disease is recommended. The celiac trunk may be engaged using a variety of catheters, including the Cobra, SoS, or Simmons. A glidewire is then advanced into the common hepatic trunk of the celiac trunk (with the image intensifier or flat panel in the posteroanterior projection), and subsequently the gastroduodenal branch. This glidewire is then used to carefully exchange the Cobra, SoS, or Simmons catheter for a more deliverable catheter such as an angled glide or Bernstein catheter. With a catheter in the gastroduodenal artery, adequate angiography of the gastroepiploic artery can be achieved.

SUMMARY

The technique of coronary angiography remains important in contemporary clinical practice. Although no didactic training can substitute for the hands-on apprenticeship obtained during general cardiology and interventional cardiology fellowships, a thorough understanding of the intellectual elements fundamental to coronary angiography outlined in this article will result in a more efficient, effective, and safe procedure for patients.

REFERENCES

1. Sones FM Jr, Shirey EK. Cine coronary arteriography. Mod Concepts Cardiovasc Dis 1962;31:735–8.
2. Amoroso G, Laarman GJ, Kiemeneij F. Overview of the transradial approach in percutaneous coronary intervention. J Cardiovasc Med (Hagerstown) 2007; 8(4):230–7.
3. Goldberg SL, Renslo R, Sinow R, et al. Learning curve in the use of the radial artery as vascular access in the performance of percutaneous transluminal coronary angioplasty. Cathet Cardiovasc Diagn 1998;44(2):147–52.
4. Louvard Y, Pezzano M, Scheers L, et al. [Coronary angiography by a radial artery approach: feasibility, learning curve. One operator's experience]. Arch Mal Coeur Vaiss 1998;91(2):209–15 [in French].
5. Jolly SS, Amlani S, Hamon M, et al. Radial versus femoral access for coronary angiography or intervention and the impact on major bleeding and ischemic events: a systematic review and meta-analysis of randomized trials. Am Heart J 2009;157(1):132–40.
6. Garrett PD, Eckart RE, Bauch TD, et al. Fluoroscopic localization of the femoral head as a landmark for common femoral artery cannulation. Catheter Cardiovasc Interv 2005;65(2):205–7.
7. Khoukaz S, Kern MJ, Bitar SR, et al. Coronary angiography using 4 Fr catheters with ACISTed power injection: a randomized comparison to 6 Fr manual technique and early ambulation. Catheter Cardiovasc Interv 2001;52(3):393–8.
8. Lefevre T, Morice MC, Bonan R, et al. Coronary angiography using 4 or 6 French diagnostic catheters: a prospective, randomized study. J Invasive Cardiol 2001;13(10):674–7.
9. Todd DM, Hubner PJ, Hudson N, et al. Multicentre, prospective, randomized trial of 4 vs. 6 French catheters in 410 patients undergoing coronary angiography. Catheter Cardiovasc Interv 2001;54(3):269–75.
10. Abhaichand RK, Louvard Y, Gobeil JF, et al. The problem of arteria lusoria in right transradial coronary angiography and angioplasty. Catheter Cardiovasc Interv 2001;54(2):196–201.
11. Barbeau GR. Radial loop and extreme vessel tortuosity in the transradial approach: advantage of hydrophilic-coated guidewires and catheters. Catheter Cardiovasc Interv 2003;59(4):442–50.
12. Valsecchi O, Vassileva A, Musumeci G, et al. Failure of transradial approach during coronary interventions: anatomic considerations. Catheter Cardiovasc Interv 2006;67(6):870–8.
13. Yokoyama N, Takeshita S, Ochiai M, et al. Anatomic variations of the radial artery in patients undergoing transradial coronary intervention. Catheter Cardiovasc Interv 2000;49(4):357–62.
14. Angelini P, Villason S, Chan AV Jr, et al. Normal and anomalous coronary arteries in humans. In: Angelini P, editor. Coronary artery anomalies. Baltimore: Lippincott Williams & Wilkins; 1999. p. 27–150.
15. West NE, McKenna CJ, Ormerod O, et al. Percutaneous coronary intervention with stent deployment in anomalously-arising left circumflex coronary arteries. Catheter Cardiovasc Interv 2006;68(6):882–90.
16. Lanzieri M, Khabbaz K, Salomon RN, et al. Primary angioplasty of an anomalous left main coronary

artery: diagnostic and technical considerations. Catheter Cardiovasc Interv 2003;58(2):185–8.

17. Cohen MG, Tolleson TR, Peter RH, et al. Successful percutaneous coronary intervention with stent implantation in anomalous right coronary arteries arising from the left sinus of valsalva: a report of two cases. Catheter Cardiovasc Interv 2002; 55(1):105–8.

18. Sapra R, Kaul U, Singh B, et al. Simplified approach of cannulating anomalously arising right coronary artery from left sinus of Valsalva. Cathet Cardiovasc Diagn 1998;45(3):346–7.

19. Qayyum U, Leya F, Steen L, et al. New catheter design for cannulation of the anomalous right coronary artery arising from the left sinus of valsalva. Catheter Cardiovasc Interv 2003;60(3):382–8.

Three-Dimensional Coronary Visualization, Part 1: Modeling

S. James Chen, PhD[a],*, Dirk Schäfer, PhD[b]

KEYWORDS

- 3D modeling • Coronary angiography • Optimal viewing
- Coronary arterial tree • Computer graphics

Despite the development of other imaging techniques, including CT and MRI, selective (ie, catheter-based) radiographic coronary angiography remains the most commonly performed method for accurate imaging of the entire coronary tree.[1-3] The technology is widely available, there are many cardiologists who are well trained in the technique and the image interpretation, the spatial and temporal resolution are unsurpassed, and the diagnostic procedure can be easily transitioned into a therapeutic procedure. In addition to providing specific anatomic information, angiography also has an important prognostic role in the identification of coronary artery disease and the associated risk for subsequent morbidity and mortality.[4-7] The number of diagnostic and therapeutic angiographic procedures has increased dramatically during the last several decades. Although it has been widely accepted and used, traditional angiography is limited by its two-dimensional (2D) representation of three-dimensional (3D) structures and the consequent imaging artifacts that impair optimal visualization. Furthermore, the techniques of image acquisition used with traditional angiography are not standardized, subjectively chosen, and highly dependent on the 3D visual skills of individual operators. Recognition of these limitations has resulted in the development of imaging techniques designed to specifically address the weaknesses of traditional angiographic techniques.

Clinicians rely on traditional 2D views or information generated from a standard radiographic imaging system to select appropriate patients for different treatments, perform catheter-based cardiovascular therapeutic or interventional procedures, and assess device-anatomy results based on the results of limited 2D quantitative analysis. Subjectively selected or standard angiographic views may produce no useful clinical information because of overlap or superimposed vessels on the angiograms. Suboptimal images may lead to mistakes, complications, and suboptimal results. Some patients who have complex anatomy may need twice the number of contrast injections to adequately visualize all segments of the coronary tree.

Because coronary anatomy is different among individuals and no reliable method has existed to determine the accuracy of standard angiographic views, no objective quantification of vessel foreshortening or overlap during routine coronary angiography and stent deployment exists. Three-dimensional techniques have recently been developed for clinical use to minimize the imaging limitations of 2D angiography. In addition to accurately displaying the complexities of coronary anatomy, 3D methods are capable of quantifying vessel curvature, measuring vessel segment length, and identifying the amount of radiographic foreshortening and vessel overlap in any simulated angiographic projection. This article describes

[a] Division of Cardiology, Department of Medicine, University of Colorado Denver, Anschutz Medical Campus, Leprino Building, 5th Floor, #519, 12401 E. 17th Avenue, B-132, Aurora, CO 80045, USA
[b] Philips Research Europe–Hamburg, Tomographic Imaging Systems, Roentgenstrasse 24–26, 22335 Hamburg, Germany
* Corresponding author.
E-mail address: james.chen@ucdenver.edu (S.J. Chen).

Cardiol Clin 27 (2009) 433–452
doi:10.1016/j.ccl.2009.03.004

the process and applications associated with producing a model of coronary vascular trees using only a few standard 2-D projection images from a routine coronary angiographic study.

THREE-DIMENSIONAL MODELING TECHNIQUE

Several techniques for estimating the 3D structure of coronary arteries using computer assistance have been developed.[8–13] These methods are based on the known or standard radiographic geometry of projections, placement of landmarks, or known vessel shape and on the iterative identification of matching structures in two or more views. Because the computation was designed for predefined views only, it was not likely to solve the modeling problem on the basis of two projections acquired at arbitrary and unknown relative orientations. Another method based on motion and multiple views acquired in a single-plane imaging system was proposed.[14] The motion transformations of the heart model consisted only of rotation and scaling. By incorporation of the center-referenced method and initial depth coordinates and center coordinates, a 3D skeleton of the coronary arteries was obtained. However, real heart motion during contraction and relaxation involves five specific movements: translation, rotation, wringing, accordion-like motion, and movement toward the center of the ventricular chamber. Therefore, the assumption did not correspond to the in vivo situation.

Other knowledge-based or rule-based systems were proposed for 3D modeling of coronary arteries by use of the model of a vascular network.[15–18] Because the rules and knowledge bases were organized for certain specific conditions, it was not feasible to generalize the 3D modeling on the basis of arbitrary projections. The advent of 3D angiography allows improvement in the quality and potentially safety of diagnostic and therapeutic endovascular procedures. The algorithms of 3D reconstruction using the cone-beam back-projection technique were proposed by other investigators.[19–21] Such techniques have been successfully applied for reconstructing nonmoving objects such as brain vessels in conjunction with a rapid rotational gantry system (at an acquisition rate of more than 40°/sec).[22–29] For a moving object such as the coronary vascular tree, the gantry system needs to be gated using an ECG signal to synchronize the same time phase. The 3D coronary artery images are created from a set of radiographic perspective projections acquired during a rotation of the imaging gantry around the patient by use of the technique of computerized cone-beam reconstruction.[30] Because of heart motion and the availability of only a limited number of projections (four or six), accurate reconstruction and quantitative measurement can not be achieved using those methods. Enhanced cone-beam reconstruction techniques have been developed to greatly improve the accuracy and quality of reconstructed 3D coronary arterial structures based on multiple angiograms acquired from a rapid rotational single-plane imaging system (see the article by Klein elsewhere in this issue).

The basic geometric mathematics for modeling 3D objects based on two views were proposed to allow for the determination of a 3D object structure using two projection images obtained at arbitrary and unknown orientations. Iterative techniques based on nonlinear equations and optimization theory were proposed for determining the solutions that characterize two views for motion analysis.[31] The results may be suboptimal if the initial conditions are chosen for a location that is beyond the proper solution space. Other analytical-based algorithms required at least eight corresponding image points in the two projections for determining the 3D position by solving a set of linear equations.[32–35] In the practical situation, however, an input image error of more than one pixel (1 pixel = 0.03 mm) in the image intensifier (17 cm × 17 cm) may result in 3D position deviations of 10 cm or more. Hence, optimal estimation has been explicitly investigated. Several two-step approaches were proposed for an optimal estimation of 3D structures based on maximum-likelihood and minimum-variance estimation.[36–40] Preliminary estimates that were computed using the linear algorithm were used as initial estimates for the process of optimal estimation. The new, recently developed C-arm imaging system is able to rapidly rotate around patients while acquiring a series of images. The 3D coronary arterial model can then be created by using more than two projection views.[41–43] However, accurate segmentation of arteries in multiple images is a crucial process and is time consuming as well, especially when a manual or interactive editing process is required. Among all the existing techniques, none has ever been applied to directly facilitate in-room clinical procedures because of the large computational cost or inadequate representation format for advanced quantitative analysis.

Basic 3D Modeling Techniques Using Two Angiographic Views

A typical on-line 3D modeling technique was proposed to accurately generate an image of the entire coronary arterial tree based on two views acquired from routine angiograms at arbitrary orientation, without the need of a calibration object, and using a single-plane imaging system.[44,45] In this method, an optimization algorithm was used to minimize the image-point and vector-angle errors in both views, subject to the constraints derived from the intrinsic parameters of the single-plane or biplane imaging system that was used. Using five or more corresponding object points in two views, the optimal estimate of the transformation in the form of a rotational matrix (R) and a translational vector can be obtained that characterizes the position and orientation of one view relative to the other. The initial solution to the optimization process is calculated on the basis of the intrinsic single-plane imaging parameters that were used. The first in-room 3D modeling of a patient-specific coronary arterial tree was performed in 1997 while the patient was lying on the table-bed in the cardiac catheterization laboratory.

Either two contrast injections for conventional acquisition or one contrast injection for rotational acquisition in a single-plane imaging system, or one contrast injection for standard acquisition in a biplane imaging system can be used to acquire a pair of angiograms associated with two different viewing angles. Each angiographic view is defined by the selected gantry orientation in terms of the left or right anterior oblique (RAO or LAO) angle and the caudal or cranial (CAUD or CRAN) angle with respect to the iso-center to which the gantry arm rotates. The gantry information, accompanying the acquired images, is automatically recorded, including focal-spot to image-intensifier distance, field of view (eg, 5-, 7-, or 9-inch mode), and gantry orientation. Generally, the process for 3D modeling of the coronary arterial tree consists of four major steps, as described in the following sections.

Image acquisition and selection
The table-bed may be moved or panned during the acquisitions in single-plane imaging systems,

which commonly happens in a routine angiographic study so that the projections of the whole coronary system can be enclosed by the scope of the image intensifier. These images are acquired at 15 or 30 frames per second in each view, with an ECG signal simultaneously recorded. The acquisition time of each frame is automatically superimposed with the associated ECG signal and displayed on the console to facilitate image selection and review, as shown in **Fig. 1**. With the acquired two angiographic sequences, a pair of cine images containing eight frames (at 15 frames/sec acquisition rate) or 15 frames (at 30 frames/sec acquisition rate) are chosen that correspond to the same or a close acquisition time (eg, end-diastole) in the cardiac cycle.

Segmentation of the 2D arterial tree and vessel feature extraction
As the result of vessel overlap, crossing, and a poor signal-to-noise ratio in angiograms, the existing automatic vessel segmentation or tracking techniques can only allow for assessment of the severity of arterial segment narrowing or a limited number of vessels instead of the complete arterial structures. To remedy this problem, a reliable semiautomatic segmentation system that uses a curve-based deformation technique is adopted to identify the entire 2D arterial tree on the pair of angiographic images.[45] The required user interaction in the identification process involves the indication of a series of points inside the lumen of each artery in the angiogram and results in several curves as the initial estimate of the vessel centerlines, as shown in **Fig. 2A**. At the next step, a filter is applied to the image to allow for identification of those pixels that have the minimum local intensity inside the lumen (see **Fig. 2A**). These points define the actual vessel centerline points (but not the continuous centerline itself). The final continuous centerline is generated by aligning the initially identified user-generated centerline toward the filter-derived centerline

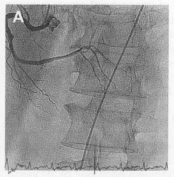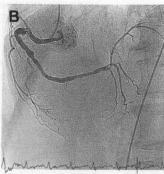

Fig. 1. (*A*) First selected angiographic view, in which the first image corresponding to the fifth R-wave of the cardiac cycle and the subsequent seven images at the LAO-CRAN view will be transferred. (*B*) Second selected angiographic view (ie, deep LAO-CRAN view), in which the image acquired at the seventh R-wave of a different cardiac cycle along with the subsequent seven images is transferred.

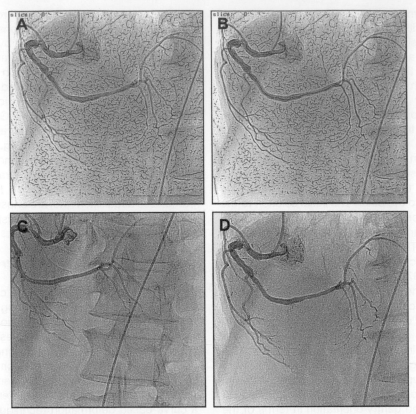

Fig. 2. (A) An example of interactively identified vessel centerlines (*green curves*) on the right coronary artery side branches that served as initial vessel centerlines and were superimposed on the derived image forces in terms of "valley" points (*red segments*). (B) The resultant vessel centerlines were aligned with the actual median lines of the artery and overlaid on the image forces after the end-of-deformation process. (C and D) The vessel features including the vessel centerline lines (*yellow curves*), bifurcation points (*blue dots*), and diameters (*short red segments*) were extracted on the pair of angiograms.

points based on a deformation model,[46,47] as shown in **Fig. 2**B. Vessel features, including bifurcation points, directional vectors at individual bifurcations, diameters, and centerline points of each artery, are extracted from the pair of angiograms that were used to facilitate the calculation of transformation and the subsequent modeling process, as shown in **Fig. 2**C, D.

Calculation of the transformation defining the spatial relationship of two views

In the single-plane imaging system used, the gantry angulations associated with different views are always recorded and accompany the acquired image file. However, a transformation that is directly calculated using the recorded gantry angles may not accurately define the spatial relationship between the two views because of images that may be acquired nonsimultaneously from two different cardiac cycles and because of table panning or movement during the acquisitions, as shown in **Fig. 3**A. Although such a directly calculated transformation cannot truly

characterize the two views, the resultant estimate is generally good enough to serve as an initial guess in the nonlinear minimization process for obtaining an optimal solution. With the initial solution calculated using gantry angles, the global minimum resulting from the nonlinear optimization can be guaranteed because the initial estimate is close to the actual solution. On the basis of the initial solution, the final accurate transformation can be calculated from an objective function by using minimization of image-point errors in terms of the square of Euclidean distance between the 2D input data and the projection of calculated 3D data points, and by using directional vector errors between the 2D vessel directional vectors and the projection of calculated 3D vessel directional vectors, as shown in **Fig. 3**B.

Calculation of the skeleton of the coronary arterial tree

On the basis of the epi-polar theory, the calculated transformation is used to establish *initial* point correspondences between each pair of 2D vessel

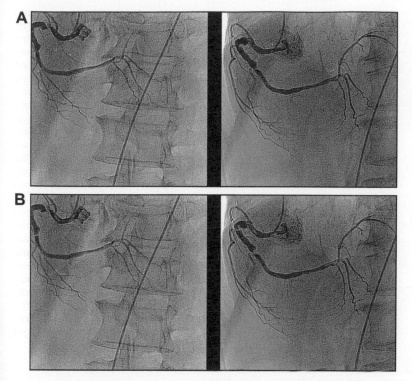

Fig. 3. (*A*) Calculated 3D bifurcation points projected to the same angiographic views used for extraction of the 2D bifurcation points (*red dots*), based on the initial transformation derived from the two viewing angles. (*B*) Final transformation was determined after minimization of the distances between the projected 3D and extracted 2D bifurcation points and the angles between the projected 3D and 2D directional vectors in both views.

centerlines by finding the intersection between the epi-polar line and vessel centerline curve (**Fig. 4**A). When the epi-polar line is "tangential" to the 2D vessel centerline curve, there will be multiple intersection points (ie, the centerline curve and epi-polar line are superimposed), and the calculated results can be heavily influenced by a small error in the 2D centerline position. To overcome the problem, a refinement process that uses the minimization algorithm[48] for segment-to-segment matching is performed. Results in the *final* point correspondences are shown in **Fig. 4**B. By use of the correspondence relationship and transformation, the 3D morphologic structures of the coronary arterial tree can be computed.[45] The resultant vessel lumen of the 3D arterial tree is modeled as a series of cross-sectional contours, with the surfaces filled between every two consecutive contours calculated using the identified 2D diameters at the second step for rendering the approximated morphology of an artery, as shown in **Fig. 4**C, D.

More than 1000 cases of left and right coronary arterial trees, saphenous vein grafts (SVGs), left internal mammary artery (LIMA) grafts, and pulmonary arterial trees have been processed based on the on-line 3D modeling techniques. In **Fig. 5**A, angiograms of an anomalous coronary artery (ACA) show where the ostium of the left coronary arterial tree comes from the proximal site of the

right coronary arterial tree. A 3D model of an ACA tree is illustrated in **Fig. 5**B. The 3D models of an SVG to the obtuse marginal (OM) branch and a LIMA graft to the left anterior descending artery (LAD), shown in **Fig. 5**D, F, were generated from the corresponding pairs of images in **Fig. 5**C, E, respectively. The accuracy of 3D length measurement was confirmed to be within an average root mean-square (RMS) of 3.5% error, using eight different pairs of angiograms of an intracoronary 105-mm guide wire with eight radiopaque markers of 15 mm interdistance. The accuracy of similarity between the additional computer-generated projections compared with the actual acquired views was demonstrated with the average RMS errors of 3.09 mm and 3.13 mm in 20 left coronary artery (LCA) and 20 right coronary artery (RCA) cases, respectively.[45]

Dynamic 3D Modeling Technique Using One Pair of Cineangiograms

Coronary arteries and veins are dynamic, curvilinear structures that have a great degree of individual-to-individual variability and tortuosity. This phasic change has been shown in cell culture models to impact endothelial function. Endothelial cells subjected to oscillating stretch demonstrate altered gene expression for endothelia, growth factors, and regulators of fibrinogen.[49] Moreover,

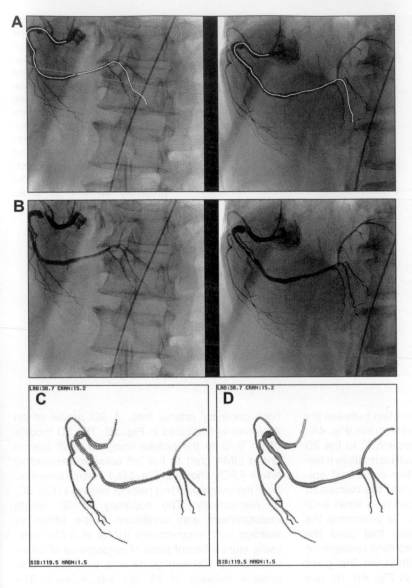

Fig. 4. (*A*) Initial correspondence of a vessel centerline point (*red dots*) in the first view (*left panel*) is established by calculating the intersection between the epi-polar line (*green line*) and the 2D vessel centerline curve in the second view (*right panel*). (*B*) Typical example of segment-to-segment matching on a pair of arterial segments to refine the vessel centerline point-to-point correspondences based on a minimization process. (*C*) Calculated skeleton structure of the right coronary arterial tree in the forms of 3D vessel centerlines (*blue lines*) and associated cross-sections (*short red segments*). (*D*) Surface-based graphic rendering technique is used to display the 3D right coronary artery tree (*pink*) and the catheter (*light blue*).

clinical events such as restenosis appear to be accelerated at areas of cyclic curvature change, which are called flexion areas.[50] Thus, geometric description of human coronary arteries represents a potentially useful method for understanding both the natural and treatment history of coronary artery disease.

In the cardiovascular arena, percutaneous catheter-based interventional (ie, therapeutic) procedures include a variety of coronary interventions, such as atherectomy and the placement of metal stents, radiation-emitting catheters, devices to trap embolized atherosclerotic debris, and pacing electrodes in the coronary venous system. These procedures use 2D radiographic-based imaging as the sole or the major imaging modality for procedure guidance and quantification of key parameters. Dynamic variations of coronary vascular curvilinearity have been very difficult to study because coronary angiographic imaging that is used clinically represents vascular structures in a 2D format. Therefore, a quantitative description of coronary geometry and motion is required both for the mathematical modeling of arterial mechanics and for the evaluation and performance of a variety of current and emerging therapeutic procedures.[51]

The dynamic 3D reconstruction technique can be used to accurately generate moving coronary arterial trees throughout the cardiac cycle based on two sequences of cineangiograms acquired from a biplane or single-plane imaging system.[48] This method consists of five major steps: (1) acquisition of two angiogram sequences based on

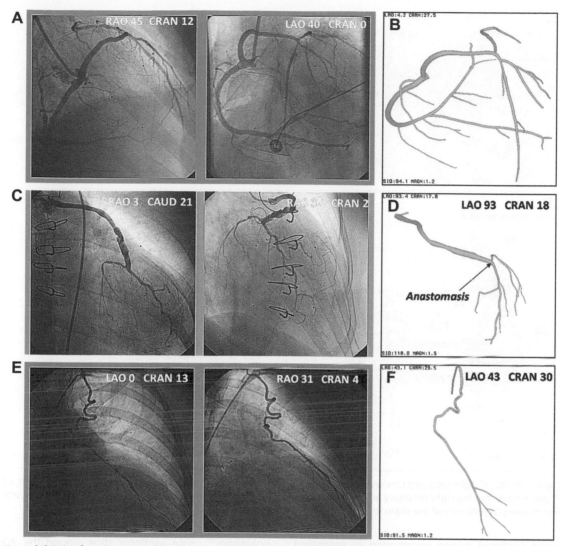

Fig. 5. (*A*) Pair of angiograms of anomalous coronary arteries. (*B*) Generated 3D model of the anomalous coronary arterial trees. (*C*) Pair of angiograms for an OM graft. (*D*) Generated 3D model of OM graft with a catheter. (*E*) Pair of angiograms for a LIMA graft. (*F*) 3D model of LIMA with a catheter.

a single-plane or biplane imaging system; (2) identification of 2D coronary arterial trees and feature extractions, including bifurcation points, vessel diameters, and vessel directional vectors in the two image sequences; (3) determination of transformation in terms of global and local transformation matrices based on the identified vessel features; (4) calculation of moving 3D coronary arterial trees based on the transformations and extracted vessel features; and (5) establishment of temporal correspondence with smoothness constraints.

Two typical examples of pairs of right and left coronary cineangiograms acquired between end-diastole (ED) and end-systole (ES) using a single-plane imaging system are shown in **Fig. 6**A and

Fig. 7A, respectively. The dynamic 3D modeling results of temporal correspondences, including six time frames for the RCA tree, are illustrated in **Fig. 6**B, C. Similarly, the 3D dynamic result for the LCA tree with the LAD and left circumflex (LCX) arteries is shown in **Fig. 7**B, C. The curved arrows represent the motion trajectories of major arteries moving from ED to ES.

Multiple View Modeling

A rotational angiography acquisition typically has a duration of more than two heart beats; therefore, more than two angiographic projections can be used to generate a 3D model that typically results in increased accuracy.[41] First, a 3D centerline skeleton is derived, and in a second step, the

A

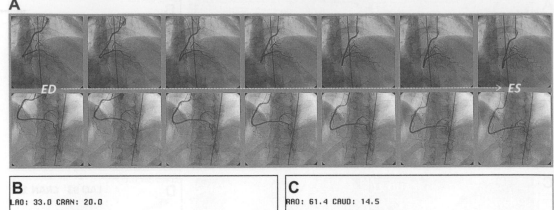

B

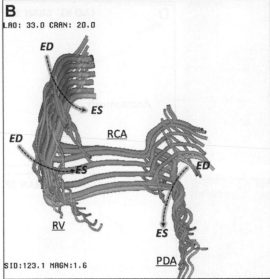

C

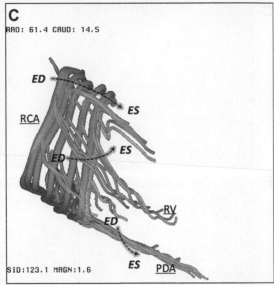

Fig. 6. (*A*) Pair of right coronary cineangiograms acquired from one half of the cardiac cycle (ie, from ED to ES. (*B, C*) A generated, moving right coronary arterial tree visualized in two angiographic views in which the arrows indicate the moving trajectories of the main RCA, posterior descending artery (PDA), and right ventricular (RV) artery.

cross-sectional lumen information is estimated from the projections. The 3D centerline may be generated by using manual,[42] semiautomatic,[43] or automatic[52] segmentation of the 2D centerlines in multiple projections and exploiting the epi-polar constraints of corresponding points.[49–51] These methods need to establish the correspondence between centerline points from different projections a posteriori, which is hampered by vessel overlap and foreshortening. The extraction of the centerline directly in 3D space using a probability map in 3D may mitigate this problem.[52]

For each 3D centerline point, corresponding 2D centerline points in every projection are now available. The endoluminal vessel borders in the projections may be determined for all these corresponding 2D centerline points by using edge detection filters combined with dynamic programming.[53,54] The various 2D cross-sections can be combined in 3D space by considering that the individual magnification factors form a convex[42] or

polygonal[55] cross-sectional slice around the 3D centerline point. Finally, the slices of neighboring centerline points are connected to build a 3D polyhedral model of the vessel or vessel segment. The process of mesh generation in 3D space is illustrated in **Fig. 8**.

Multiple-view modeling results from a rotational acquisition along a circular arc are shown in **Fig. 9**. Two hundred and ten projections were acquired during 7 seconds while the patient held his breath. The number of 3D models that can be derived from the projection data and can represent distinct cardiac phases increases with an increase in the frame rate and decreases with an increase in the heartbeat rate.[55] To ensure robust automatic 3D model generation, the heart rate should be strong enough to provide at least five projections per cardiac phase.[52] In the example of **Fig. 9**, with 30 projections and 90 heartbeats per second, 20 distinct models can be generated. The centerlines of the 3D models from three different cardiac

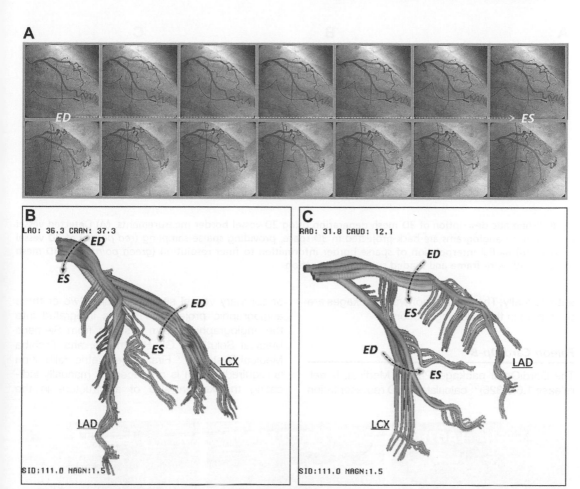

Fig. 7. (*A*) Pair of left coronary cineangiograms acquired from one half of cardiac cycle (ie, from ED to ES). (*B, C*) A generated moving left coronary arterial tree visualized in two angiographic views in which the arrows indicate the moving trajectories of the left LAD artery and the LCX artery.

phases (see **Fig. 9**D–F) are overlaid on the corresponding projections (see **Fig. 9**A–C) from similar angles. The forward-projected 3D centerline does not always coincide perfectly with the center of the vessel in the 2D angiogram because of residual nonperiodic motion. However, the lumen information for the vessel modeling is extracted from motion-corrected 2D angiograms. The vessel dynamics can be analyzed using this multiphase 3D model without the drawbacks of foreshortening and overlap that are present in dynamic 2D angiograms.

The multiple-view modeling discussed in the previous paragraphs is not restricted to rotational acquisitions along a circular arc. Modeling results obtained using projection data acquired while the C-arm rotates around two axes at the same time[56] are shown in **Fig. 10**. The trajectory (see **Fig. 10**C) passes close to that of several standard views used for diagnostic 2D angiography and can be acquired using a single injection of contrast

agent in 6.5 seconds. The angiograms have been acquired with patient breath hold at a heartbeat rate of 75 beats per minute. The projections marked by the green triangles and red diamonds on the trajectory in **Fig. 10**C have been used to generate the 3D model shown in **Fig. 10**D, whereas the red diamonds indicate the projection angles of the angiograms shown in **Fig. 10**A, B.

SURVEY ON COMMERCIALLY AVAILABLE PACKAGES

Several 3D coronary artery modeling packages are available from different companies. They are all semiautomatic in the sense that several points on the vessel of interest have to be clicked manually in two or more angiographic projection images from different gantry positions. The vessel borders in the individual 2D projections are delineated automatically and can be refined manually. Based on this user interaction, a 3D model is computed

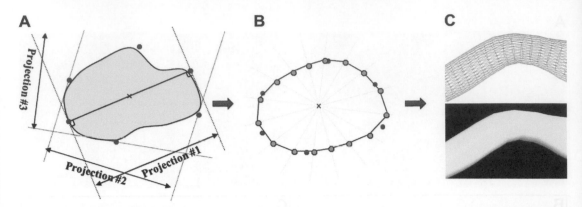

Fig. 8. Schematic description of 3D mesh generation using 2D vessel border measurements. (*A*) Detected vessel borders in 2D angiograms are back-projected in 3D space, providing sparse sampling (*red points*) of 3D vessel borders. (*B*) Radial interpolation of sparse border information to finer resolution (*green points*). (*C*) 3D mesh buildup with wire frame and shaded surface visualization.

automatically. The different software packages are presented in the following sections.

Paieon CardiOp-B

The CardiOp-B package (Paieon Medical, Israel, release 1.6.8.326)[57] calculates a 3D representation of coronary vessel segments using two or three angiographic projections and is integrated into the angiographic C-arm systems from Siemens Medical Solutions, GE Healthcare, and Toshiba Medical Systems.[57] First, a geometric calibration is required, which is produced by manually indicating the known size of a structure in the

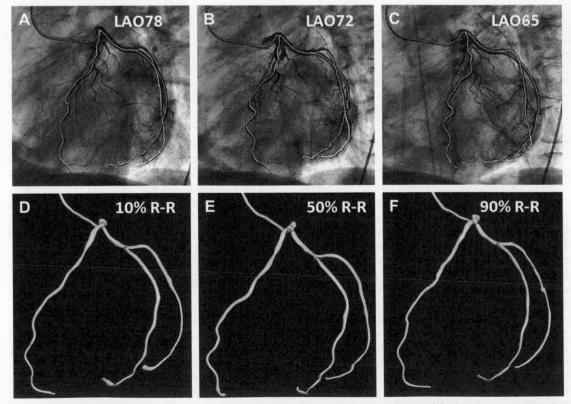

Fig. 9. Multiphase angiograms with 3D centerline overlay and corresponding 3D models. (*A–C*) Projections using circular arc acquisition from different angles and cardiac phases. (*D–F*) Multiple-view 3D models corresponding to the cardiac phases of the angiograms in *A* to *C*, with fixed viewing direction for display.

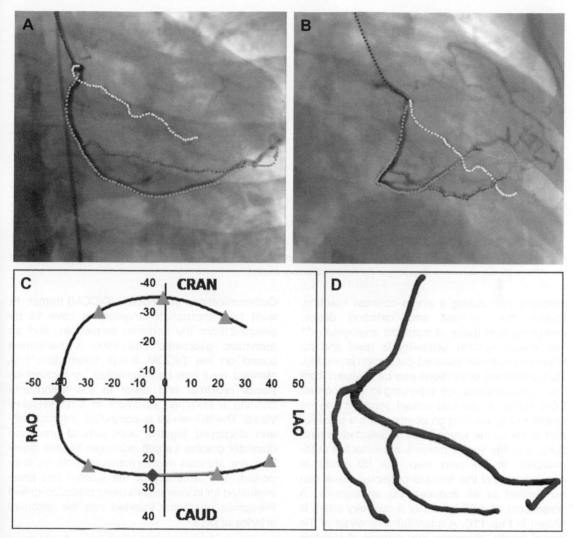

Fig. 10. (*A*, *B*) Angiograms with 3D centerline overlay acquired at the angles marked with red diamonds along the rotational dual-axis acquisition, as shown in (*C*). (*D*) Multiple-view 3D model generated from projections acquired at the angles marked with green triangles and red squares in (*C*).

projection image, either in French scale units or in millimeters. After calibration, a projection appropriate for 2D segmentation can be selected. A stenotic area can be segmented by clicking on one point in the middle of the lesion and two points that are proximal and distal to the lesion. In a second projection, three similar clicks are required. The 3D model is calculated automatically. An optimal third projection direction is suggested to further improve the model. A screenshot of a 3D model of a phantom is shown in **Fig. 11**A. Diameter, stenosis degree, and length of the vessel segment are displayed as graphs, and numbers for stenosis degree and minimum luminal diameter are given. The presented values are claimed to be accurate within ± 0.1 mm for diameter, ± 5% for length, and ± 0.4 mm^2 for

area measurements.[57] Evaluation studies indicate that length measurements are accurate,[58,59] but lumen measurements are underestimated.[59–61] The CardiOp-B package can calculate bifurcation parameters and has been used to analyze the geometric and angle changes that may occur after stent implantation in bifurcation lesions.[62]

Philips 3D-CA

The Allura 3D-CA package (Philips Healthcare, the Netherlands)[63] calculates a 3D representation of the coronary arteries using two angiographic projections from a rotational radiographic acquisition and is available with the Philips Allura C-arm family. Rotational angiography is used to acquire dynamic multiple-angle projections of the

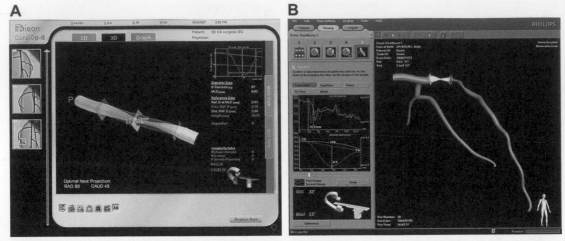

Fig. 11. (*A*) Screen shot of the CardiOp-B software showing a 3D model of a vascular phantom. (*B*) Screen shot of the Allura 3D-CA software showing a 3D coronary artery model.

coronary tree during a single-contrast injection, limiting the contrast and radiation doses, compared with those of standard angiography.[64] The known system geometry is used and no manual or catheter-assisted calibration is needed. Two consistent projections can be selected from the rotational sequence according to the recorded ECG signal. A stenotic vessel segment can be delineated by clicking on points that are proximal and distal to the lesion in both selected projections, and the vessel borders are detected automatically. In the next step, the 3D model is computed, and the forward-projected result can be verified in all acquired 2D angiograms. A screenshot of a 3D model of a coronary artery is shown in **Fig. 11**B. A quantitative analysis of the vessel length, diameter, and degree of stenosis is displayed. A color-coded optimal view map is visualized, indicating angle areas with the least amount of foreshortening of the vessel segment. Evaluation studies indicate that length measurements are accurate within 2%,[65] that the radiation and contrast doses are reduced,[66] and that optimized working views with less foreshortening can be identified compared to operator selected working views.[65,67] Bifurcation modeling is possible by adding a new vessel segment to an existing one, and by repeating this step, the whole coronary tree can be modeled.

Pie Medical CAAS QCA3D

The Cardiovascular Angiography Analysis System for 3D Quantitative Coronary Analysis (CAAS QCA3D, Pie Medical Imaging, the Netherlands)[68] can be used to calculate 3D representations from vessel segments and bifurcations from imported angiograms using the Digital Imaging and Communications in Medicine (DICOM) format. At least two appropriate angiograms have to be selected from the acquired sequences, and an automatic geometric calibration is performed based on the DICOM image information.[61] A stenotic area can be segmented by clicking on points proximal and distal to the lesion and defining a common landmark in both selected views. The 3D model is computed automatically and displayed together with luminal area and diameter graphs. Length, minimum luminal diameter, and stenosis degree measurements are supported. The accuracy of the system has been evaluated for in vivo studies using precision-drilled Plexiglass phantoms inserted into the coronary arteries of pigs.[61]

APPLICATIONS USING 3D CORONARY MODELING
Current Clinical Application

For a complex intervention, patients receive substantial amounts of radiation and contrast material during diagnostic and interventional procedures. Much of the radiation and contrast material use is linked to the operator choosing views that are adequate for diagnosis and intervention. This traditional trial-and-error method provides views (or optimal views) in which overlap and foreshortening are minimized, but only in terms of the subjective, experience-based judgment of the angiographer.[44,45] The 3-D models derived from any of the methods described provide the clinician with the ability to rotate the model into all simulated angiographic views. This functionality allows the clinician to observe how different views display the patient's anatomy and coronary lesions without exposing the patient to additional radiation and contrast media. Optimal views, that is, angiographic views that display the region of interest without overlap from surrounding vessels and with foreshortening of the segment, can be derived by either rotating the model on a computer screen or using computer assistance to solve these imaging tasks. Early studies of optimal view strategy[13] only focused on minimization of vessel foreshortening relative to a single arterial segment, but then the optimal-view strategy on the basis of minimization of both vessel overlap and foreshortening was proposed.[44,45] When this article was written, more than 60 instances of 3D modeling had been performed in-room to assist in interventions while patients were lying on the table-bed during cardiac catheterization.[51]

Advanced Applications

Coronary artery analysis for assessment of stent conformability

Implanted stents may result in a permanent modification of the curvilinearity of the artery. It has been hypothesized that the frequently observed straightening effect of stents implies an uneven distribution of forces within the arterial wall, potentially augmenting the injury reaction of the vessel wall and thereby increasing the rate of restenosis. The impact of stent-induced arterial straightening during cardiac contraction is also unknown but clearly is greater at ES when arteries are normally more tortuous, shortened, and flexed. Therefore, a 3D arterial image can be generated before and after stent implantation, based on the 3D modeling technique such that the shape change can be assessed to quantify the degree of vessel straightening effect. A typical example of 3D RCA models with stenotic lesions at ED and ES is shown in **Fig. 12**A (or see Video 1, available in the on-line version of this article at: http://www.cardiology.theclinics.com). Three-dimensional models of the RCA tree with straightened arterial segments after stent implantation are shown in **Fig. 12**B (or see Video 2, available in the on-line version of this article at: http://www.cardiology.theclinics.com/). The amount of vessel straightening can be easily quantified by comparing the shape change of the 3D RCA models at the ED and ES, as shown in **Fig. 12**C, D (also see Videos 3 and 4, respectively, available in the on-line version of this article at: http://www.cardiology.theclinics.com/).

Coronary vein analysis for resynchronization therapy

There has been recent enthusiasm for left ventricular or biventricular pacing as therapy for patients who have advanced congestive heart failure to improve the patient's ejection fraction by enhancing the synchronization of myocardial contraction (ie, cardiac resynchronization therapy).[69–74] Coronary sinus implantation is currently the most popular method.[73,74] Its main advantage is a totally transvenous approach. The lead, which is inserted into the subclavian vein, is advanced to the left ventricular free wall by way of a venous tributary of the coronary sinus. However, the difficulties posed by this method are significant in view of the pronounced anatomic variation in the coronary venous anatomy from patient to patient and the reliance on the use of traditional fluoroscopic images to guide navigation and placement of pacing leads in the coronary venous system. Currently, the presence, diameter, angulation, and tortuosity of veins as visualized using 2D retrograde venography are used to determine their acceptability for the placement of a lead in a predetermined location. By use of prolonged, routine angiographic acquisition, coronary venograms can be easily acquired, as shown in **Fig. 13**A, B. Then 3D models of coronary venous trees at ED and ES can be created, as shown in **Fig. 13**C, D (or see Video 5, available in the on-line version of this article at: http://www.cardiology.theclinics.com/), including models of the coronary sinus, great cardiac vein, anterior interventricular vein, and several major side branches such as the middle cardiac vein, posterior vein, and left marginal vein. Using the 3D vein models, the anatomic information such as the 3D diameter of the coronary sinus, take-off angles of side branches, and individual pathway lengths originating from the coronary sinus to individual side branches can be quantified to facilitate the determination of an optimal implantation site.

Coronary artery and vein analysis for transvenous mitral annuloplasty

A novel technique of transvenous mitral annuloplasty has been introduced for reduction of mitral valve regurgitation. Such a procedure currently relies on 2D radiographic-based imaging as the sole or the major imaging modality for guidance and quantification of key parameters. Three-dimensional coronary venous and nearby arterial anatomy must be visualized and quantified for planning and performing the intervention. In **Fig. 14**A, B, a pair of routine coronary cineangiograms containing the delayed venous phase was acquired based on a single-plane imaging system and with patient breath holding. The 3D coronary arterial and venous trees consisting of the major and secondary vessels were created at the ED

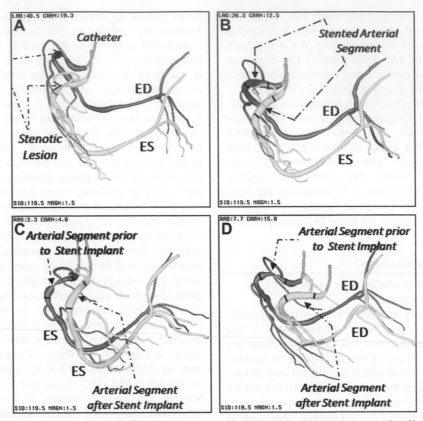

Fig. 12. (*A*) 3D models of RCA trees generated from two pairs of angiographic images at ED (*pink*) and ES (*yellow*) time points at which a tight stentotic lesion occurred at the proximal RCA segment. (*B*) The 3D models of RCA trees generated from another two pairs of angiographic images at ED (*pink*) and ES (*yellow*) time points after stent implantation on the lesion site. The shape change between the 3D arterial segments before and after stent implantation is illustrated at the ES (*C*) and ED (*D*) time points.

and ES, as shown in **Fig. 14**C, D, respectively (or see Video 6, available in the on-line version of this article at: http://www.cardiology.theclinics.com/). The geometric evaluation of the venous system includes measurements of length, diameter, radius of curvature, and the take-off angle of the side branch, and a stereoscopic rendering to inspect the spatial relationship of the major venous pathway from the great cardiac vein to the anterior interventricular vein (ie, crossover or parallel to each other) relative to its adjacent companion artery. The 3D anatomy, morphologic variation, and spatial relationship of the coronary artery and vein can be accurately assessed using angiographic data. This information can be used for patient selection, device sizing, and optimal placement of a coronary venous device for mitral annulus repair.

Intracardiac lead deformation for fatigue and fracture analysis

The implantable cardioverter-defibrillator (ICD) is an electronic device to detect and stop serious ventricular arrhythmias and restore a normal heartbeat in people who are at high risk for sudden death. According to the American College of Cardiology, more than 80,000 Americans currently have an ICD. The ICD is usually implanted below the collarbone just beneath the skin. Cardiac leads are the conduits through which ICDs regulate the heartbeat with electrical impulses.[75,76] The proximal end of the lead is connected to the ICD device, and the distal end is threaded into the heart through a vein located near the collarbone. The tip of each lead is positioned in direct contact with the tissue inside the heart. Although it is pliable, the lead is not designed to tolerate excessive flexing, bending, or tension. This could cause structural weaknesses, conductor discontinuity, or dislodgment of the lead. If the leads for ICDs become ineffective as the result of fracture, certain serious problems may occur, such as nondectection of an arrhythmia, oversensing of the heart rate, or inadequate delivery of converting energy. It is very important to identify the sites of maximum stress for lead motion or to localize the

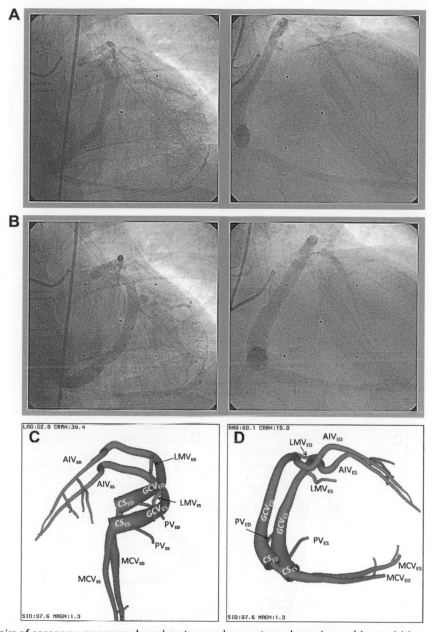

Fig. 13. Two pairs of coronary venograms based on two prolong antegrade angiographic acquisitions at the ED (*A*) and the ES (*B*) time points. (*C, D*) Generated 3D models of coronary venous trees consisting of several major side branches visualized at two different viewing angles. AIV, anterior interventricular vein; CS, coronary sinus; GCV, great cardiac vein; LMV, left marginal vein; MCV, middle cardiac vein; PV, posterior vein.

site of potential lead fracture in vivo for lead design and testing. On the basis of a pair of cineangiographic images, as shown in **Fig. 15**A (or see Video 7, available in the on-line version of this article at: http://www.cardiology.theclinics.com/), in vivo, dynamic 3D models of the lead throughout one half of the cardiac cycle (ie, from ED to ES) can be generated, as shown in **Fig. 15**B. Based on the 3D lead models, the motion trajectory and bending radii of the lead can be quantified, as

illustrated in **Fig. 15**C, D (also see Videos 8 and 9, respectively, available in the on-line version of this article at: http://www.cardiology.theclinics. com/). The 3D modeling technique and quantitative analysis allow for quantitative assessment of unique patient-specific characteristics of an implanted cardiac lead. The 3D motion pattern of cardiac lead can be used to improve the design and manufacture of more reliable and safer cardiac leads.

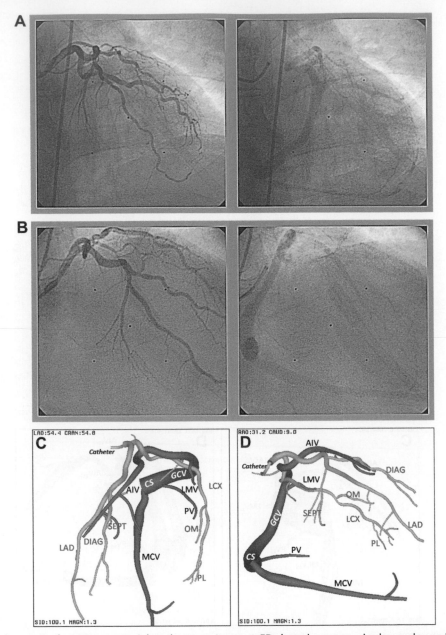

Fig. 14. Angiograms of coronary arterial and venous trees at ED, based on one, single, prolonged, antegrade angiographic acquisition for the first view (*A*) and the second view (*B*). (*C, D*) The generated 3D models of coronary arterial and venous trees consisting of major side branches show the complex spatial relationship at two different viewing angles. AIV, anterior interventricular vein; CS, coronary sinus; DIAG, diagonal branch; GCV, great cardiac vein; LAD, left anterior descending artery; LCX, left circumflex artery; LMV, left marginal vein; MCV, middle cardiac vein; OM, obtuse marginal artery; PL, posterior lateral artery; PV, posterior vein; SEPT, septal branch.

DISCUSSION AND SUMMARY

The 3D models generated using the modeling approaches are based on extraction of centerline and diameter data from 2D angiographic images. Therefore, the morphology of vessel lumens can only be approximated. As a result, plaque with irregular shapes or eccentric lesions in arteries will not be truly portrayed based on the 3D modeling technique. Other imaging modalities such as CT and magnetic resonance angiography have the ability to provide volumetric data.

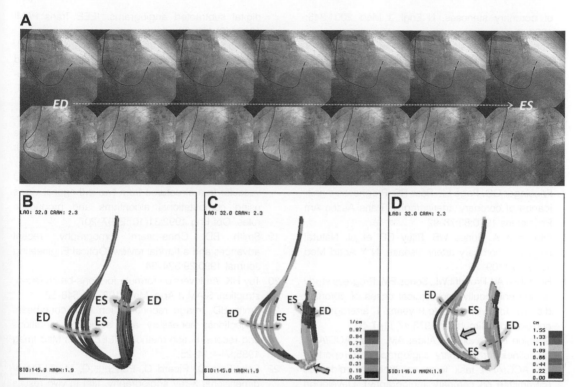

Fig. 15. (*A*) Pair of cineangiograms of a temporal intracardiac lead placed in the outflow track of the right ventricle, acquired at half of the cardiac cycle. (*B*) Generated 3D models of a moving intracardiac lead in which the arrows indicate the motion pathways of the tip and midportion of the lead during half of the cardiac cycle. (*C*) Color coded leads illustrate the translational movements with respect to the position of the lead at the ED (*purple*) during half of the cardiac cycle in which the largest translation occurred at the midportion of the lead (*orange arrow*). (*D*) In vivo bending radii of the lead in terms of curvatures during half of the cardiac cycle are color coded on the surfaces in which the maximal bending area is indicated by an orange arrow.

However, these technologies have limited use for studying conformational changes in the artery caused by stainless-bare-metal-based or metal-alloy-based implanting devices because of artifacts in signals or heating problems. Despite this limitation, the authors believe that the 3D modeling technique can be easily used to create in vivo and patient-specific 3D vascular models, in patients with or without implanted coronary devices, based on 2D angiographic images acquired from a conventional or more-advanced imaging system.

There is no doubt that there is clinical value in the first step of transforming 2D projection images into a 3D model of the patient's arterial tree. There is further value in performing a quantitative analysis of key geometric features from the 3D models. Finally, decision-making support can provide assistance to the physician in solving imaging tasks such as the determination of an optimal projection view of a coronary artery lesion needing treatment. Each of these three important processes must occur in the clinical environment where actions must be made within minutes of image acquisition.

Using the 3D modeling technique, the authors expect that more quantitative tools will be developed and implemented for clinical use that are applicable today but also generic enough to allow application to future interventions, other vascular trees, and future imaging modalities. Specifically, these novel, patient-specific, four-dimensional (ie, 3D morphology and one-dimension in time-varying space) vascular and implanted device models, along with the advanced quantitative tools, will be adopted routinely to improve procedure outcomes and enhance patient safety during percutaneous, catheter-based interventions.

APPENDIX: SUPPLEMENTARY MATERIAL

Supplementary data associated with this article can be found in the on-line version, at: doi: 10.1016/j.ccl.2009.03.004.

REFERENCES

1. Kim WY, Danias PG, Stuber M, et al. Coronary magnetic resonance angiography for the detection

of coronary stenoses. N Engl J Med 2001;345: 1863–9.

2. Achenbach S, Giesler T, Ropers D, et al. Detection of coronary artery stenoses by contrast-enhanced, retrospectively electrocardiographically gated, multislice spiral computed tomography. Circulation 2001;103:2535–8.

3. Achenbach S, Moshage W, Ropers D, et al. Value of electronbeam computed tomography for the noninvasive detection of high-grade coronary artery stenoses and occlusions. N Engl J Med 1998;339: 1964–71.

4. Friesinger GC, Page EE, Ross RS. Prognostic significance of coronary arteriography. Trans Assoc Am Physicians 1970;83:78–92.

5. Oberman A, Jones WB, Riley CP, et al. Natural history of coronary artery disease. N Y Acad Med 1972;48:1109–25.

6. Bruschke AV, Proudfit WL, Sones FM. Progress study of 590 consecutive nonsurgical cases of coronary disease followed for 5 to 9 years. I. arterographic correlations. Circulation 1973;47:1147–53.

7. Scanlon PJ, Faxon DP, Audet AM, et al. ACC/AHA guidelines for coronary angiography: a report of the ACC/AHA task force on practice guidelines (committee on coronary angiography). Developed in collaboration with the society for cardiac angiography and interventions. J Am Coll Cardiol 1999; 33(6):1756–824.

8. Kim HC, Min BG, Lee TS, et al. 3D digital subtraction angiography. IEEE Trans Med Imaging 1982;MI-1: 152–8.

9. Potel MJ, Rubin JM, Mackay SA, et al. Methods for evaluating cardiac wall motion in 3D using bifurcation points of the coronary arterial tree. Invest Radiol 1983;18:47–56.

10. Parker KL, Pope KL, van Bree R, et al. 3D reconstruction of moving arterial beds from digital subtraction angiography. Comput Biomed Res 1987;20:166–85.

11. Kitamura K, Tobis JM, Sklansky J. Estimating the 3D skeletons and transverse areas of coronary arteries from biplane angiograms. IEEE Trans Med Imag 1988;MI-7:173–87.

12. Pellot CP, Herment A, Sigelle M, et al. A 3D reconstruction of vascular structures from two X-ray angiograms using an adapted simulated annealing algorithm. IEEE Trans Med Imag 1994;13(1):49–60.

13. Dumay ACM, Reiber JHC, Gerbrands JJ. Determination of optimal angiographic viewing angles: basic principles and evaluation study. IEEE Trans Med Imag 1994;13(1):13–24.

14. Nguyen TV, Sklansky J. Reconstructing the 3D medial axes of coronary arteries in single-view cineangiograms. IEEE Trans Med Imag 1994;13(1):48–60.

15. Stansfield S. ANGI: a rule-based expert system for automatic segmentation of coronary vessels from digital subtracted angiograms. IEEE Trans PAMI 1986;8(2):188–99.

16. Garreau M, Coatrieux JL, Collorec R, et al. A knowledge-based approach for 3D reconstruction and labeling of vascular networks from biplane angiographic projections. IEEE Trans Med Imag 1991; 10(2):122–31.

17. Fessler JA, Macovski A. Object-based 3D reconstruction of arterial trees from magnetic resonance angiograms. IEEE Trans Med Imag 1991;10(1): 25–39.

18. Liu I, Sun Y. Fully automated reconstruction of 3D vascular tree structures from two orthogonal views using computational algorithms and production rules. Opt Eng 1992;31(10):2197–207.

19. Smith BD. Cone-beam tomography: recent advances and a tutorial review. Optical Engineering Journal 1990;29:524–34.

20. Tuy HK. An inversion formula for cone-beam reconstruction. SIAM J Appl Math 1983;43:546–52.

21. Smith BD. Image reconstruction from cone-beam projections: necessary and sufficient conditions and reconstruction methods. IEEE Trans Med Imag 1985;MI-4:14–25.

22. Saint-Felix D, Picard C, Ponchut C, et al. Three-dimensional X-ray angiography: first in vivo results with a new system. SPIE: Medical Imaging: Image capture, formatting, and display, Newport Beach. California 1897;90–98:1993.

23. Anxionat R, Bracard S, Macho J, et al. 3D angiography: clinical interest—first applications in interventional neuroradiology. J Neuroradiol 1998;25: 251–62.

24. Grass M, Koppe R, Klotz E, et al. Three-dimensional reconstruction of high contrast objects using C-arm image intensifier projection data. Comput Med Imaging Graph 1999;23(6):311–21.

25. Moret J, Kemkers R, Beek J, et al. 3D rotational angiography: clinical value in endovascular treatment. Medicamundi 1998;42(3):8–14.

26. Koppe R, Klotz E, Op de Beek J, et al. 3D vessel reconstruction based on rotational angiography. Proceedings CAR '95, Berlin, June 21–24,101–7, 1995.

27. Koppe R, Klotz E, Op de Beek J, et al. Digital stereotaxy/stereotactic procedures with C-arm based rotational angiography. Proceedings CAR '96, Paris, 17–22, 1996.

28. Koppe R, Klotz E, Op de Beek J, et al. 3D reconstruction of cerebral vessel malformations based on rotational angiography (RA). Proceedings CAR '97, Berlin, 145–51, 1997.

29. Kemkers R, Op de Beek J, Aerts H, et al. 3D-rotational angiography: first clinical application with use of a standard Philips C-arm system. Proceedings CAR '98, Tokyo, 182–7, 1998.

30. Rougee A, Picard C, Sanit-Felix D, et al. 3D coronary arteriography. Int J Card Imaging 1994;10:67–70.

31. Roach JW, Aggarwal JK. Determining the movement of objects from a sequence of images. IEEE Trans PAMI 1980;2:554–62.

32. Longuet-Higgins HC. A computer algorithm for reconstructing a scene from two projections. Nature 1981;293(10):133–5.

33. Tsai RY, Huang TS. Uniqueness and estimation of 3D motion parameters of rigid objects with curved surfaces. IEEE Transon PAMI 1984;6(1):13–27.

34. Metz CE, Fencil LE. Determination of three-dimensional structure in biplane radiography without prior knowledge of the relationship between the two views: theory. Med Phys 1989;16(1):45–51.

35. Hoffmann KR, Metz CE, Chen Y. Determination of 3D imaging geometry and object configurations from two biplane views: an enhancement of the Metz-Fencil technique. Med Phys 1995;22(8):1219–27.

36. Weng J, Huang TS, Ahuja N. A two-step approach to optimal motion and structure estimation. Proc IEEE Workshop Computer Vision 1987;87:355–7.

37. Weng J, Ahuja N, Huang T. Closed-form solution and maximum likelihood: a robust approach to motion and structure estimation. Proc IEEE Conf Computer Vision and Pattern Recognition 1988;381–6.

38. Weng J, Huang TS, Ahuja N. Motion and structure from two perspective views: algorithms, error analysis and error estimation. IEEE Transon PAMI 1989; 11:451–76.

39. Weng J, Ahuja N, Huang TS. Optimal motion and structure estimation. IEEE Trans on PAMI 1993; 15(9):864–84.

40. Chen SYJ, Metz CE. Improved determination of biplane imaging geometry from two projection images and its application to 3D reconstruction of coronary arterial trees. Med Phys 1997;24(5): 633–54.

41. Sprague K, Drangova M, Lehmann G, et al. Coronary x-ray angiographic reconstruction and image orientation. Med Phys 2006;33(3):707–18.

42. Movassaghi B, Rasche V, Grass M, et al. A quantitative analysis of 3D coronary modeling from two or more projection images. IEEE Trans Med Imag 2004;23(12):1517–31.

43. Blondel C, Malandain G, Vaillant R, et al. Reconstruction of coronary arteries from a single rotational X-ray projection sequence. IEEE Trans Med Imag 2006;25(5):653–63.

44. Chen SYJ, Carroll JD. On-line 3D reconstruction of coronary arterial tree based on a single-plane imaging system. Circulation 1997;96(8):308.

45. Chen SYJ, Carroll JD. On-line 3D reconstruction of coronary arterial tree for optimization of visualization strategy using a single-plane imaging system. IEEE Trans Med Imag 2000;19(4):318–36.

46. Kass M, Witkin A, Terzopoulos D. Snakes: active contour models. International Journal of Computer Vision 1988;1:321–31.

47. Williams DJ, Shah M. A fast algorithm for active contours. International Journal of Computer Vision 1992;55:14–21.

48. Chen SYJ, Carroll JD. Kinematic and deformation analysis of 4-D coronary arterial trees reconstructed from cine angiograms. IEEE Trans Med Imag 2003; 22(6):710–21.

49. Davies PF, Tripathi SC. Mechanical stress mechanisms and the cell. Circ Res 1993;72:239–45.

50. Stein PD, Hamid MS, Shivkumar K, et al. Effects of cyclic flexion of coronary arteries on progression of atherosclerosis. Am J Cardiol 1994;73: 431–7.

51. Chen SYJ, Carroll JD, Messenger JC. Quantitative analysis of reconstructed 3D coronary arterial tree and intracoronary devices. IEEE Trans Med Imag 2002;21(7):724–40.

52. Jandt U, Schäfer D, Rasche V, et al. Automatic generation of 3D coronary artery centerlines using rotational X-ray angiography. Proc Soc Photo Opt Instrum Eng 2007;6510:65104Y1–8.

53. Figueiredo M, Leitiio J. A nonsmoothing approach to the estimation of vessel contours in angiograms. IEEE Trans Med Imag 1995;14(1):162–72.

54. Sonka M, Winniford M, Collins S. Robust simultaneous detection of coronary borders in complex images. IEEE Trans Med Imag 1995;14(1):151–61.

55. Jandt U, Schäfer D, Grass M, et al. Automatic generation of time resolved motion vector fields of coronary arteries and 4D surface extraction using rotational X-ray angiography. Phys Med Biol 2009; 54:47–66.

56. Horisaki T, Iinuma K, Bakker N. Feasibility evaluation of dual axis rotational angiography (XperSwing) in the diagnosis of coronary artery disease. Medica Mundi 2008;52(2):11–3.

57. Available at: http://www.paieon.com. Accessed April 29, 2009.

58. Gollapudi R, Valencia R, Lee S, et al. Utility of three-dimensional reconstruction of coronary angiography to guide percutaneous coronary intervention. Catheter Cardiovasc Interv 2007;69:479–82.

59. Gradaus R, Mathies K, Breithardt G, et al. Clinical assessment of a new real time 3D quantitative coronary angiography system: evaluation in stented vessel segments. Catheter Cardiovasc Interv 2006; 68:44–9.

60. Tsuchida K, van der Giessen W, Patterson M, et al. In vivo validation of a novel three-dimensional quantitative coronary angiography system (CardiOp-B): comparison with a conventional two-dimensional system (CAAS II) and with special reference to optical coherence tomography. EuroIntervention 2007;3:100–8.

61. Ramcharitar S, Daeman J, Patterson M, et al. First direct in vivo comparison of two commercially available three-dimensional quantitative coronary

angiography systems. Catheter Cardiovasc Interv 2008;71:44–50.

62. Dvir D, Marom H, Assali A, et al. Bifurcation lesions in the coronary arteries: early experience with a novel 3-dimensional imaging and quantitative analysis before and after stenting. Eurointervention 2007;3:95–9.

63. Available at: http://www.healthcare.philips.com. Accessed April 29, 2009.

64. Maddux J, Wink O, Messenger J, et al. Randomized study of the safety and clinical utility of rotational angiography versus standard angiography in the diagnosis of coronary artery disease. Catheter Cardiovasc Interv 2004;62:167–74.

65. Garcia JA, Chen J, Hansgen A, et al. Rotational angiography (RA) and three-dimensional imaging (3DRA): an available clinical tool. Int J Cardiovasc Imaging 2007;23:9–13.

66. Koester R, Grass M, Begemann P, et al. Initial results of three-dimensional rotational coronary angiography. March 29–April 1, Paper 2515-4. Chicago, USA: SCAI–ACCi2 Conference; 2008.

67. Green NE, Chen SY, Hansgen AR, et al. Angiographic views used for percutaneous coronary interventions: a three-dimensional analysis of physician-determined vs. computer-generated views. Catheter Cardiovasc Interv 2005;64:451–9.

68. Available at: www.piemedicalimaging.com. Accessed April 29, 2009.

69. Izutani H, Quan KJ, Biblo LA, et al. Biventricular pacing for congestive heart failure: early experience in surgical epicardial versus coronary sinus lead placement. Heart Surg Forum 2003;6(1):E1–6.

70. Abraham WT. Late-breaking clinical trials: results from late-breaking trial sessions at ACC 2001. J Am Coll Cardiol 2001;38:604–5.

71. Cazeau S, Leclercq C, Lavergne T, et al. Effects of multisite biventricular pacing in patients with heart failure and intraventricular conduction delay. N Engl J Med 2002;344:873–80.

72. Kuhlkamp V. Initial experience with an implantable cardioverter-defibrillator incorporating cardiac resynchronization therapy. J Am Coll Cardiol 2002; 39:790–7.

73. Leclereq C, Cazeau S, Le Breton H, et al. Acute hemodynamic effects of biventricular DDD pacing in patients with end-stage heart failure. J Am Coll Cardiol 1998;32:1825–31.

74. Touiza A, Etienne Y, Gilard M, et al. Long-term left ventricular pacing: assessment and comparison with biventricular pacing in patients with severe congestive heart failure. J Am Coll Cardiol 2001; 38:1966–70.

75. C Butter, E Meisel, J Tebbenjohanns,et al. Transvenous biventricular defibrillation halves energy requirements in patients. Circulation 2001;104:2533–8

76. Alonso C, Leclercq C, d'Allonnes FR, et al. Six-year experience of transvenous left ventricular lead implantation for permanent biventricular pacing in patients with advanced heart failure: technical aspects. Heart 2001;86:405–10.

Three-Dimensional Coronary Visualization, Part 2: 3D Reconstruction

Gert Schoonenberg, MSc[a,b,*], Anne Neubauer, PhD[c],
Michael Grass, PhD[d]

KEYWORDS

- 3D coronary angiography • Catheterization
- Tomographic reconstruction • Cardiac gating • Motion

The use of angiographic X-ray systems to provide CT-like tomographic images is called three-dimensional (3D) X-ray tomography. In the interventional domain, this technique was initially introduced for neurovascular imaging, where the 3D reconstruction of contrast agent (CA)-enhanced vascular structures from rotational X-ray projections led to improved visualization of abnormalities.[1] As in the neurovascular domain, tomographic coronary artery reconstruction adds a new dimension to two-dimensional (2D) angiographic-projection imaging, which remains the predominant workhorse for percutaneous coronary interventions (PCI). The incorporation of 3D information provides a variety of advantages. These include the accurate visualization and sizing of vessel segments, lesions, and bifurcations in 3D, the presentation of 3D roadmap information, the ability to use or predict any projection view for intervention guidance, even those which were not acquired, and the calculation of optimal viewing directions.

Three-dimensional coronary reconstruction is based on the acquisition of rotational projection sequences with or without electrocardiogram (ECG) triggering. In contrast to CT, the rotational projections (ie, a series of 2D coronary angiograms)

can be used themselves for diagnosis, while the reconstruction processing is used to transform the acquired data into volume information. As a result, a 3D-volume dataset is generated to represent the X-ray absorption of the object of interest in each voxel position. Consequently, the entire volume dataset consists of the CA-enhanced vascular structures, as well as other objects with X-ray absorption capability surrounding the vessels. This positions 3D coronary reconstruction in the domain of tomographic imaging, in contrast to manual or automatic modeling techniques (please see the article by Chen and Schäefer in this issue.), which generate binary (vessel versus no vessel) 3D-object representations, typically in the form of centerlines with diameter information.

Three-dimensional coronary tomography using interventional X-ray systems is a new application in medical imaging and is currently under development. The original concept of tomographic imaging of the human heart is almost as old as that of X-ray-based tomography itself.[2] Starting in the 1990s, the first coronary reconstructions were performed using fast tomosynthesis-acquisition strategies.[3] The problem of cardiac motion was addressed and solved with a complex

[a] Department of Cardiovascular Innovation, Business Unit Cardio/Vascular X-Ray, Philips Healthcare, Veenpluis 4-6, 5680 DA Best, The Netherlands
[b] Division Biomedical Imaging and Modeling, Department of Biomedical Engineering, Eindhoven University of Technology, Den Dolech 2, 5600 MB Eindhoven, The Netherlands
[c] Philips Research North America, 345 Scarborough Road, Briarcliff Manor, NY 10510, USA
[d] Philips Technologie GmbH Forschungslaboratorien, Röntgenstr. 24-26, D-22335 Hamburg, Germany
* Corresponding author. Department of Cardiovascular Innovation, Business Unit Cardio/Vascular X-Ray, Philips Healthcare, Veenpluis 4-6, 5680 DA Best, The Netherlands.
E-mail address: gert.schoonenberg@philips.com (G. Schoonenberg).

Cardiol Clin 27 (2009) 453–465
doi:10.1016/j.ccl.2009.03.006

hardware setup to freeze the motion of the coronaries. Over time, the focus shifted toward the development of 3D coronary angiography using existing cardiac X-ray angiography systems, where the cardiac motion problem is approached via advanced reconstruction methods. A continuous flow of new reconstruction schemes has been introduced in recent years, which resulted in steadily improved image quality for 3D coronary angiography. Therefore, 3D coronary angiography is now positioned at the cusp between technical and clinical research.

This article reviews the strategies, challenges, and results of 3D coronary tomography. The potential role of 3D coronary reconstruction in PCI and some tools and clinical findings based on current implementation are also discussed.

DATA ACQUISITION

Three-dimensional reconstruction of coronary arteries from X-ray projections requires the acquisition of angiographic data along a circular short-scan trajectory (ie, 180°–220°) during continuous CA injection (**Fig. 1**). Usually, this is achieved via a power injector filling the coronary arteries at a flow rate of 1 mL/sec to 2 mL/sec throughout the acquisition (please see the article by Klein and Garcia in this issue). In addition, the vessel tree of interest needs to be well iso-centered, such that all relevant segments are present in the 2D images throughout the acquisition. In principle, the object to be reconstructed should be stationary during the image acquisition, though this is obviously not achievable in cardiac imaging. While breathing and patient movement can be minimized by appropriate setup and instruction, the cardiac motion of the heart must be tackled with strategies such as gating (see "Cardiac gating and phase selection strategies") or motion compensated reconstruction techniques (see "Motion-compensated Reconstruction Methods").

The data acquisition duration and angular coverage are limited by both spatial constraints

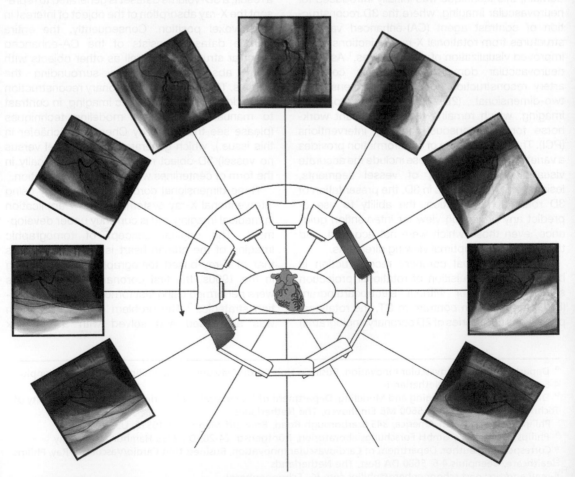

Fig. 1. Schematic illustration of the short-scan or 200° rotational acquisitions for tomographic 3D X-ray reconstruction.

in the clinical environment and hardware constraints of the acquisition system. Compared with the angular coverage needed for coronary modeling, as described in the article by Chen and Schäefer in this issue, the angular coverage required for reconstruction needs to be larger. Most of the rotational acquisitions for 3D coronary artery reconstruction are based on a 180° to 220° circular arc acquisition. Different start and end gantry arm positions, as well as angular speed, may be chosen. A typical example of an acquisition has a starting position of the C-arm at left anterior oblique (LAO) 120° and proceeds to right anterior oblique (RAO) 60° while rotating at 27° to 29° per second.[4] The rotational acquisitions can take between 4 and 8 seconds at frame rates from 30 Hz to 60 Hz. The estimated effective dose for a typical acquisition of 8.6 seconds at 30 Hz using a torso phantom (posterior-anterior diameter 24 cm, left-right diameter 30 cm) is 0.8 mSv, based on an estimated dose-area product with an effective dose conversion factor of 0.183 mSv/(Gy cm^2).[5]

To reconstruct the volume data from a series of images with high spatial resolution acquired from the digital-detector system, the geometric calibration of the imaging system is required before the clinical data acquisition. The strategy used for determining the geometrical parameters of the projections is presented in **Fig. 2**. Most of the calibration methods that are used for this purpose are phantom based.[6–8] The calibration should be performed periodically on an imaging system to ensure accurate 3D reconstruction for clinical application. Calibration is required approximately every 6 months or whenever hardware changes are made.

CARDIAC GATING AND PHASE SELECTION STRATEGIES

ECG-based gating techniques are well known and adopted for tomographic-based reconstruction of cardiac CT.[9] The main idea of gated reconstruction is to use only a subset of images from an acquisition, which correspond to a particular cardiac phase. To reconstruct a sharp image of the coronaries in the beating heart, projection images corresponding to the same cardiac phase need to be chosen for reconstruction,[10,11] which results in a 3D representation of the coronaries in that specific time point. This principle can be applied repeatedly to generate multiple 3D representations for different cardiac phases within one cardiac cycle, which allows the generation of 4D (3D plus time) renderings of the coronaries in the beating heart. These 3D representations for different cardiac phases have varying image quality because of the fact that the coronaries move with different speed depending on the individual rates of heart beat during image acquisition.[12] Less movement results in better image quality. Empirically, cardiac movement has the least motion at the end-systolic and late-diastolic cardiac phases, which theoretically provide the highest image quality when chosen for a gated reconstruction. Because of human variation, the exact position of these cardiac phases with respect to the detected R-peaks of the ECG signal differ between patients and need to be determined.

Optimal Cardiac Phase Determination

There are multiple methods to estimate the optimal cardiac phase for gated reconstruction.[13–16] The

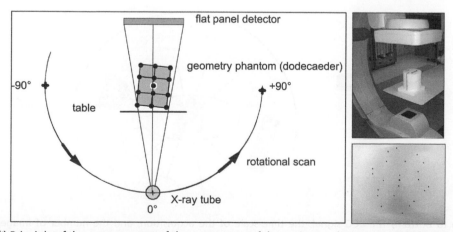

Fig. 2. (*Left*) Principle of the measurement of the parameters of the projection (geometry calibration). (*Right*) The phantom for physical geometry calibration phantom is positioned at the iso-center of the C-arm system (*upper image*) and a single projection of the geometry phantom is shown (*lower image*).

optimal cardiac phase can be determined using the ECG signal, or the image content, or both. The ECG signal measures electrical activity of the heart, which precedes contraction of the heart muscles and therefore indirectly reflects the motion of the coronaries. This simple measure can be used to select phases of the heart that are likely to have the least motion.

The cardiac phase of least motion can also be determined with the overall motion of the contrast in the projection images. Assuming the periodicity of the heart cycles is known with respect to the images of the rotational run, one can estimate the cardiac phase in which the average motion in the projection images of the rotational run is least.

Optimal Gating Window

The next step of the gating process is defining an appropriate gating window. Using just one image at the right cardiac phase for each heartbeat, so-called the "nearest neighbor gating," was the first approach used in rotational 3D coronary angiography.[10] While this represents the best opportunity for freezing the cardiac motion, the signal-to-noise ratio is severely compromised because of the low number of projections used in the reconstruction. For example, for a 7-second rotational acquisition, only five to eight images are used for reconstruction when the nearest-neighbor gating is chosen. To compensate for this, a wider gating window is used so that multiple images are taken from each heartbeat. The shape of the gating window can vary from a rectangular shape, where each chosen image contributes equally to the final reconstruction, to a half-bell shape, such that the images at the center of the gating window contribute most while those at the edges of the window contribute only slightly. Using multiple projection images around the chosen cardiac phase generally results in better-gated reconstructions. However, if the chosen window is too wide, motion artifacts will occur.[11] A schematic representation of the gating process is given in **Fig. 3**, for the example of late-diastolic gating at 70% of the cardiac cycle using a cosine-squared

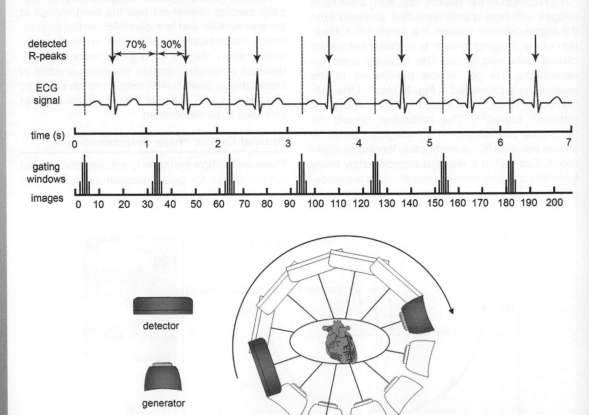

Fig. 3. (*Top to bottom*) The ECG signal, the time scale of the acquisition, and the number of images acquired including the gating windows (*vertical bars*, height indicating the relative weight), and the middle projection image of each gating window. The gating windows are given for a selected phase at 70% of the R-R interval (*dotted line* on ECG signal), with a 20% cosine-squared gating window.

gating-window shape with a width equal to 20% of the cardiac cycle in a 7-second rotational X-ray acquisition. Here, a total of 35 out of the 200 measured projections are selected for the reconstruction process (five projections per gating window).

THREE-DIMENSIONAL CORONARY RECONSTRUCTION METHODS

Mainly, two different reconstruction approaches have been applied to 3D-rotational coronary angiography so far. Direct inversion methods, as 3D cone-beam filtered-back projection, are usually based on Feldkamp's original approach.[17] While this was originally developed for ideal circular (360°) trajectories, modifications for short-scan (180°–220°) trajectories designed for angiographic X-ray systems have been introduced and successfully applied in the area of neuroradiology.[18] The application of cardiac gating, which drastically reduces the number of input images for reconstruction, to this approach results in a compromise between image quality and signal-to-noise ratio.[10,11,15] Iterative reconstruction methods can overcome these limitations by incorporating a-priori assumptions in the reconstruction process.[4] The improvement on the final image quality is counter balanced by additional computational overhead. These may result in an increase of reconstruction time that hinders clinical workflow.

Both reconstruction approaches can be combined with motion-compensation methods to tackle the problem of cardiac motion. The motion compensation can be performed either on the projection or in the 3D volume and helps to compensate for the reduction in input image data because of gating. A comparative presentation of the different approaches is given in the subsequent subsections.

Gated Reconstruction Methods

The unique requirements of interventional imaging, which differ substantially from noninvasive imaging techniques, have led to the development of reconstruction strategies that seek to provide rapid results with no user interaction. The different coronary artery reconstruction methods that have been proposed in the literature vary according to several criteria (see **Table 1**), including acquisition differences (need for ECG input and breath-holding) as well as image-processing differences. Those that use gating to minimize motion artifacts[4,10,15] can be generally classified according to whether they adopt physiologic gating from the ECG signal alone or an image intensity-based measurement to estimate motion on a per image basis. Hansis and colleagues[4] and Rasche and colleagues[10] use retrospective gating on the ECG recorded during image acquisition to select a subset of images for 3D reconstruction. Because

Table 1
Comparison of different coronary artery reconstruction strategies

	Rasche[10,14]	Lehmann[15]	Hansis[16,22]	Blondel[13]	Schäfer[11]
ECG required?	Y	N	Y	N	Y
Breath-hold required?	Y	Y	Y	N	Y
Rotational acquisition protocol	From LAO 120° to RAO 60° in 7–8 sec.	Rotation over 200° in 4.5 sec.	From LAO 120° to RAO 60° in 7–8 sec.	From LAO 120° to RAO 200° in 3–5 sec.	From LAO 120° to RAO 60° in 7–8 sec.
Optimal phase determination	Image quality criteria	SIC1[a]	Line integral method	N/A	N/A
Motion-compensation type	N/A	N/A	2D	3D	3D
Reconstruction technique	3D back-projection (FDK[b])	3D back-projection (FDK[b])	START[c]	ART[d]	3D back-projection (FDK[b])

[a] SIC: Superior-inferior component of the weighted centroid.
[b] FDK: Method developed by Feldkamp, David, and Kress.
[c] START: Simultaneous thresholding algebraic reconstruction technique.
[d] ART: Algebraic reconstruction technique.

the individual heart rates might be very different during the acquisition, it becomes important to identify the adequate width of gating window and correct phase to perform 3D reconstruction. Initial attempts tried to use specific cardiac phases that were predicted to have the least motion physiologically, such as end-diastole. However, heart-rate irregularity and variability between patients can produce suboptimal results using a fixed phase for all other patients. Rasche and colleagues[14] use image-quality criteria to classify the intensity values of the vessels over the reconstructed images. In their technique, the best cardiac phase with minimal motion was assumed to have a narrower intensity distribution because of the lack of blurring (**Fig. 4**). Blondel and colleagues[13] use a line-integral method that has less computational effort. The raw projection images before performing a reconstruction were used such that the phase with the least motion can be selected without investing reconstruction time for each phase. Specifically, each horizontal line in each projection is integrated to create one vertical line, which represents the location of the bulk of the intensity. When all the vertical line components from the other projections were placed together, the resultant picture illustrated the shifting of

contrast during the heart beat. This image can then be used to estimate the phase during which the gating window should be positioned with the least blurring effect caused by motion. This method is feasible because the axis of the rotation of the C-arm system is approximately in the same direction as the main vector of both, the cardiac and respiratory motion. An example reconstruction generated using this technique is shown in **Fig. 5**.

Lehmann and colleagues[15] used a technique very similar to the line-integral method described above to replace the ECG signal as an image-based gating technique. There have been attempts to apply similar approaches in the cardiac CT arena.[19] In the publication by Lehmann and colleagues, this approach was termed the "superior-inferior" component of the centroid, which calculates the vertical motion in the projections using an intensity sum. After plotting this motion vector, they use first and second derivatives to estimate the velocity and trigger points of the motion, respectively, to automatically determine the rest phase. Results of using this technique for reconstruction showed that it may slightly improve small-vessel visualization when compared with ECG gating alone, while also not

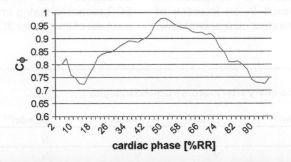

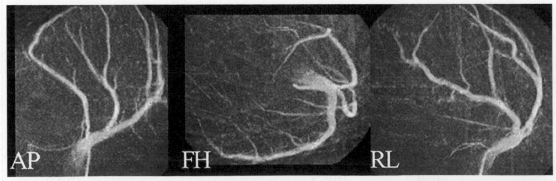

Fig. 4. (*Top*) Image-quality measure (c_ω) computed from reconstructions at different cardiac phases. (*Bottom*) Pig left coronary artery reconstructed at the optimal phase (maximum c_ω) displayed as maximum intensity projection from three different viewing directions. *From* Rasche V, Movassaghi B, Grass M, et al. Automatic selection of the optimal cardiac phase for gated three-dimensional coronary X-ray angiography. Acad Radiol 2006;13:630–40; with permission.

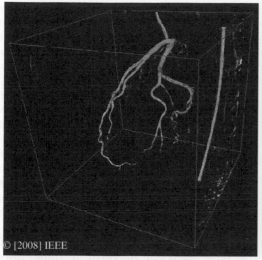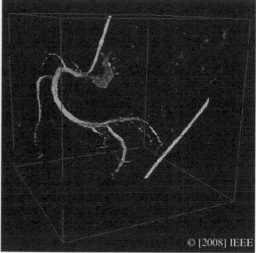

Fig. 5. Optimal phase reconstructions of left and a right coronary arterial trees from human datasets based on an iterative reconstruction method with sparse data constraint and nearest-neighbor gating presented as a volume rendering. *From* Hansis E, Schäfer D, Dössel O, et al. Evaluation of iterative sparse object reconstruction from few projections for rotational coronary angiography. IEEE Trans Med Imaging 2008;27(11):1548–55; with permission. Copyright © 2008 IEEE.

requiring the simultaneous acquisition of an ECG signal during data acquisition.

Motion-compensated Reconstruction Methods

While gating techniques seek to solve the problem of cardiac motion via selection of projection images associated with the same motion stage, motion-compensation techniques try to estimate the cardiac motion in order to actively incorporate it into the tomographic reconstruction. To accomplish this goal, the motion-vector field, which describes the geometric transformation of a heart during the cardiac cycle, must be determined. Two different motion compensation approaches have been developed for 3D coronary reconstruction, namely 2D- and 3D-motion compensation.

Obviously, the heart—and therefore the coronaries—moves in 3D throughout the cardiac cycle. Therefore, to accurately account for the movement, a 3D representation of the motion-vector field is required (an example is shown in **Fig. 6**). Blondel and colleagues[13] and Schäfer and colleagues[11] demonstrate a 3D motion-compensation approach used in combination with iterative and filtered-back projection-reconstruction methods, respectively. Because motion-compensated reconstruction requires the knowledge of the motion-vector field before reconstruction, both techniques use the 3D-centerline information throughout multiple cardiac phases of the cardiac-vessel tree to determine the motion-vector

field.[20,21] As a consequence of the limited motion information provided by tracking the vessel centerlines alone, the motion-vector field needs to be extrapolated throughout the 3D-volume space before the reconstruction process is performed.

Theoretically, all projections acquired during a rotational coronary angiography can be used for reconstruction to generate the final 3D data,

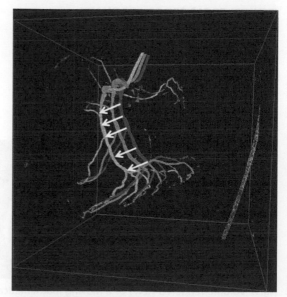

Fig. 6. Reconstructions of a right coronary arterial tree from a rotational X-ray sequence showing the spatial difference in the 3D location at three different cardiac phases. *White arrows* indicate changing location due to cardiac motion.

460 Schoonenberg et al

provided that the motion-vector field can be determined with sufficient accuracy for all cardiac phases. Thus, this strategy can significantly increase the overall signal-to-noise ratio while also reducing artifacts caused by gating. **Fig. 7** shows reconstructions using an increasing number of projection images from left to right, as well as a reference reconstruction. Practically, a combined gated- and motion-compensated approach provides a compromise, as the accurate estimation of the motion-vector field throughout different cardiac phases remains challenging.

Alternatively, 2D projection-based motion compensation can also be applied for the case of 3D coronary reconstruction.[22] Using a reconstruction created in a reference phase (eg, using gated reconstruction) and a method for 3D centerline detection, the reference-vessel centerlines are forward projected to all 2D images acquired inside the gating window. Here, the forward-projected 3D centerlines are compared with the actual detected 2D centerlines and the motion is corrected by warping the actual projection to the reference-motion state. Though the 2D images only represent a projection of the complete object, 2D motion compensation works well because the coronary arteries represent a small portion of the image with little overlapping signal from the chest. Overlapping vessels or catheters within the field of view violate this guideline and need to be handled by a more sophisticated process.

CLINICAL TOOLS FOR 3D CORONARY RECONSTRUCTION

The 3D reconstruction in conjunction with gating using optimal phase selection, motion compensation, based on a rotational X-ray angiography acquisition create a volumetric dataset of a realistic 3D left or right coronary artery tree. These datasets can be viewed and further processed in different ways. An intuitive way to investigate the data is to render the dataset on a computer screen using general volume-rendering approaches, such as maximum intensity projections (MIP), endoviews, or planar reformatting projection. Volume rendering is a visualization technique to display a 3D dataset on a screen while partially conserving the 3D information, (see **Figs. 5** and **6**). An MIP is a visualization technique that projects only the voxels with maximum intensity along a line through the dataset on the screen (see **Fig. 4**). Another volume rendering approach is called "endoview," which allows for investigation of the interior of reconstructed structures by placing a virtual camera inside the dataset. **Fig. 8C** shows an endoview rendering of a coronary artery bifurcation. A cross-sectional reformatting plane displays a single slice of the dataset in a plane perpendicular to the vessel centerline, which provides a simulated intravascular-ultrasound view of the vessel lumen. **Fig. 8B** shows a cross-section of the coronary artery displayed in **Fig. 8A**, with the automatically calculated minimum and maximum diameters labeled.

In addition to visualization of 3D coronary arteries, other clinical tools are available to analyze the volumetric dataset and provide clinical information. For example, the operator can select a coronary segment of interest for quantitative analysis by clicking a proximal and distal point on a coronary to start an automated segmentation process. This process will identify the centerline of the vessel segment, as well as the border of the contrast-filled vessel segment. This facilitates the execution of two powerful clinical tools: optimal viewing angle selection and 3D quantitative coronary analysis (QCA). Because the exact 3D location and shape of the vessel centerline is known, the optimal C-arm position for viewing the

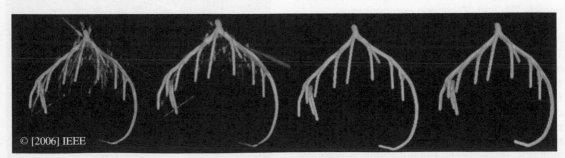

© [2006] IEEE

Fig. 7. Volume-rendered views of a moving mathematical coronary artery phantom reconstructed from a circular arc trajectory. (*Left to right*) Nearest-neighbor gated reconstruction, gated reconstruction with 20% gating-window width, motion-compensated reconstruction, reference reconstruction of the static phantom from all projections. *From* Schäfer D, Borgert J, Rasche V, et al. Motion compensated and gated cone beam filtered back projection for 3D rotational angiography. IEEE Trans Med Imaging 2006;25(7):898–906; with permission. Copyright © 2006 IEEE.

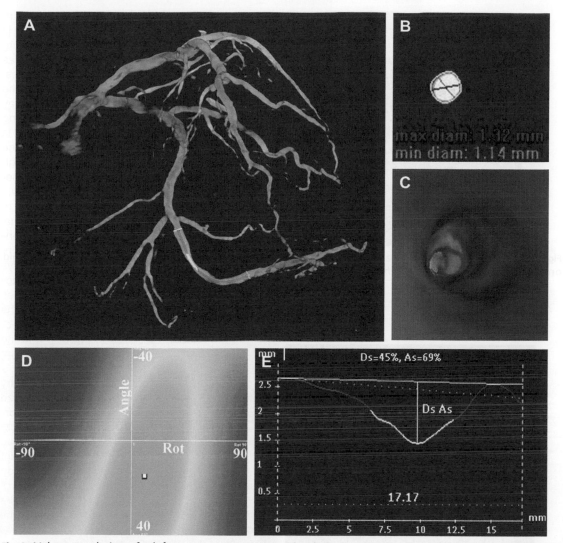

Fig. 8. Volume rendering of a left coronary artery tree with a lesion in the obtuse marginal branch defined (*A*) (*blue and yellow*), cross-sectional view (*B*), and endoview (*C*) of the lesion; optimal view map of the defined segment (*D*), and 3D-QCA (*E*) showing the degree of narrowing.

segment with least foreshortening can be calculated. **Fig.** 8D shows the amount of foreshortening for each position of the C-arm and highlights the view, such that the segment of interest has the least amount of foreshortening.[23,24] This allows the cardiologist to navigate the C-arm to that position to perform the intervention with an optimal view of the segment. Three-dimensional QCA of the vessel segment provides a diameter and surface profile along the vessel centerline that allows, for example, analyzing the reference diameter and surface area proximal and distal to a lesion, as well as the length and percent stenosis of the lesion in 3D (**Fig.** 8E).

In addition to tools for analyzing a specific vessel segment of interest, other tools exist that can help physicians to use the 3D reconstruction to plan and assist subsequent interventions. For example, there is functionality available termed "follow C-arc," which allows the operator to physically rotate the C-arm to a new position while the vessel reconstruction rotates on the screen simultaneously. This allows the interventionist to select a new working view with a sneak preview, without the need for additional contrast or radiation. Another way to use the 3D reconstructions is to overlay or forward-project the reconstructed vessels on top of a live cine or fluoroscopy image during a procedure (**Fig.** 9). This gives an indication of where the vessels are located without injecting contrast. This can improve visual guidance and navigation, while potentially reducing CA usage.

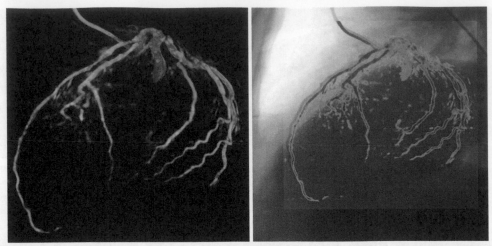

Fig. 9. Example of overlay functionality showing a gated 3D reconstruction of a left coronary artery (*left*) overlaid onto a live fluoroscopy image (*right*) during contrast injection.

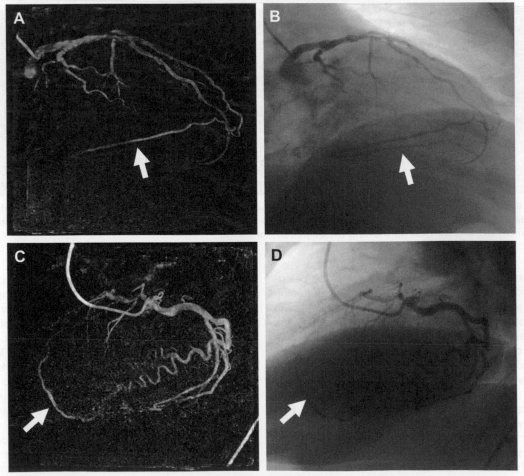

Fig. 10. MIPs from a 3D volume of two different clinical cases (*A* and *C*), which show left-to-right collateral flow (*arrows*) reconstructed using START, compared with the angiogram from the same angulation (*B* and *D*).

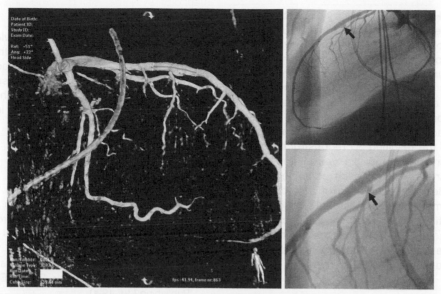

Fig. 11. In-room reconstruction (*left*) from a patient with a left-anterior descending coronary artery (LAD) pseudoaneurysm (*arrows* on angiograms on *right*), shown as volume rendering.

CLINICAL CASES

To demonstrate the current clinically achievable image quality for 3D tomographic coronary imaging during interventions, a number of datasets, which have been acquired at the University of Colorado in Denver, Colorado, are presented and discussed. The patient data were acquired using an extended-contrast injection into the coronary arteries to allow 180° rotational angiography for 3D reconstruction. Software has been developed that allows for 3D reconstruction of these data right after completion of the image acquisition, without the need of user interaction.

Fig. 10 shows two cases where the right coronary artery was nearly totally occluded and substantial left to right collateralization was visible on the raw 2D-projection images. These collateral vessels, which are quite small and slowly opacified, represent a challenge for any reconstruction

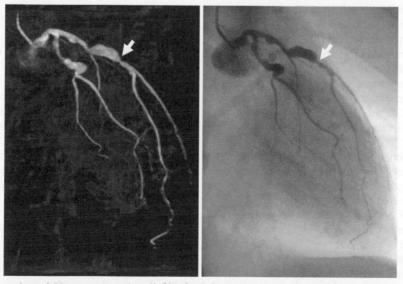

Fig. 12. Forward-projected 3D reconstruction (*left*) of a left coronary artery tree showing extensive aneurysmal segments as well as a tight LAD stenosis (*arrow*). The 2D angiogram acquired from the same angulation is also shown (*right*).

technique. However, the results indicate that these vessels are faithfully reconstructed using the aforementioned reconstruction strategy. **Fig. 11** shows a case in which a pseudoaneurysm was created during a primary coronary angioplasty procedure. The 3D reconstruction clearly shows the defect and was used in-room to help determine its positioning to aid in choosing a clinical course of action. In **Fig. 12**, both the raw angiograms and the resulting 3D reconstruction show large aneurysms in multiple vessels of the left coronary artery, one of which contained a tight stenosis. Because positioning of a stent next to a wide diameter aneurysm is challenging, the 3D reconstruction, when used in conjunction with tools such as 3D QCA and live overlay, may provide the operator with additional information that can aid in sizing and placement.

CONCLUSION AND DISCUSSION

The use of tomographic 3D coronary reconstruction based on rotational angiographic X-ray systems has evolved in recent years from a purely technical research arena toward an in-room clinical tool during PCIs. Continuous improvements in volume image quality characterized by decreasing motion artifact and increasing signal-to-noise ratio and vessel sharpness can be observed. In parallel, utilities and tools have been developed that permit lesion assessment through 3D QCA. Three-dimensional coronary visualization and quantitative analysis, such as optimal working-view selection for specific vessel segments and improved guidance via overlay functionality or follow C-arc, create a new paradigm shift for the traditional PCI. Multiple reconstructions from different cardiac phases result in a 4D representation of the coronaries to analyze coronary motion and can be potentially used for 4D-overlay functionality to serve as a time-varying roadmap.

Two current limitations of this technique are the integration of the acquisition strategy, which includes rotational acquisition with iso-centering, breath-hold, and long-contrast injection into the interventional procedure, and the high computer-processing time for generating the volume datasets. The latter becomes a more significant issue when multiple reconstructions, consisting of multiple 3D-volume datasets at different cardiac phases, are desired. However, if the resulting 3D or 4D data provide substantially useful information to the physician, neither of the issues mentioned above are likely to inhibit this technology in the long term.

ACKNOWLEDGMENTS

The authors would like to acknowledge John Carroll, MD, and the Cardiac Catheterization Laboratory at the University of Colorado Denver, for data presented in the clinical cases section. We also gratefully acknowledge Eberhard Hansis (Philips Research Europe) for his help in the preparation of **Fig. 7**.

REFERENCES

1. Kemkers R, Op de Beek J, Aerts H, et al. 3D rotational angiography: first clinical application with use of a standard Philips C-arm system. In: Proceedings of the CAR Conference. Tokyo: June 24–27;1998. p. 182–7.
2. Webb S. From watching the shadows: the origins of radiological tomography. Bristol, England: IOP Publishing Ltd; 1990.
3. Stiel G, Stiel L, Klotz E, et al. Digital flashing tomosynthesis: a promising technique for angiocardiographic screening. IEEE Trans Med Imaging 1993; 12(2):314–21.
4. Hansis E, Schäfer D, Dössel O, et al. Evaluation of iterative sparse object reconstruction from few projections for rotational coronary angiography. IEEE Trans Med Imaging 2008;27(11):1548–55.
5. Betsou S, Efstathopoulos EP, Katritsis D, et al. Patient radiation doses during cardiac catheterization procedures. Br J Radiol 1998;71:634–9.
6. Rougee A, Picard C, Trousset Y, et al. Geometrical calibration for 3D X-ray imaging. In: Proceedings of the SPIE Conference: Image Capture, Formatting and Display. Newport Beach: February 14;1993. p. 161–9.
7. Koppe R, Klotz E, Op de Beek J, et al. 3D vessel reconstruction based on rotational angiography. In: Proceedings of CAR Conference. Berlin: June 21–24;1995. p. 101–7.
8. Koppe R, Klotz E, Op de Beek J, et al. Digital stereotaxy/stereotactic procedures with C-arm based rotation-angiography. In: Proceedings of CARS Conference. Paris: June 26–29;1996. p. 17–22.
9. Kachelriess M, Kalender W. Electrocardiogram correlated image reconstruction reconstruction from subsecond multi-slice spiral computed tomography scans of the heart. Med Phys 1998;25: 2417–31.
10. Rasche V, Movassaghi B, Grass M, et al. Three dimensional X-ray coronary angiography in the porcine model: a feasibility study. Acad Radiol 2006;13:644–51.
11. Schäfer D, Borgert J, Rasche V, et al. Motion compensated and gated cone beam filtered back projection for 3D rotational angiography. IEEE Trans Med Imaging 2006;25(7):898–906.

12. Vembar M, Garcia M, Heuscher D, et al. A dynamic approach to identifying desired physiological phases for cardiac imaging using multi-slice spiral CT. Med Phys 2003;30(7):1683–93.

13. Blondel C, Malandain G, Vaillant R, et al. Reconstruction of coronary arteries from a single rotational X-ray projection sequence. IEEE Trans Med Imaging 2006;25(5):653–63.

14. Rasche V, Movassaghi B, Grass M, et al. Automatic selection of the optimal cardiac phase for gated three-dimensional coronary X-ray angiography. Acad Radiol 2006;13:630–40.

15. Lehmann G, Holdsworth D, Drangova M. Angle-independent measure of motion for image based gating in 3D coronary angiography. Med Phys 2006;33(5):1311–20.

16. Hansis E, Schäfer D, Dössel O, et al. Automatic optimum phase point selection based on centerline consistency for 3D rotational coronary angiography. IJCARS 2008;3(3–4):355–61.

17. Feldkamp LA, Davis LC, Kress JW. Practical cone-beam algorithms. J Opt Soc Am 1984;6:612–9.

18. Grass M, Koppe R, Klotz E, et al. Three-dimensional reconstruction of high contrast objects using C-arm image intensifier projection data. Comput Med Imaging Graph 1999;23:311–21.

19. Kachelriess M, Sennst D, Maxlmoser W, et al. Kymogram detection and kymogram correlated image reconstruction from sub-second spiral computed tomography scans of the heart. Med Phys 2002; 29:1489–503.

20. Blondel C, Vaillant R, Malandain G, et al. 3D tomographic reconstruction of coronary arteries using a pre-computed motion vector field. Phys Med Biol 2004;49:2197–208.

21. Jandt U, Schäfer D, Rasche V, et al. Automatic generation of time resolved motion vector fields of coronary arteries and 4D surface extraction using rotational X-ray angiography. Phys Med Biol 2009; 54:47–66.

22. Hansis E, Schäfer D, Dössel O, et al. Projection based motion compensation for gated coronary artery reconstruction from rotational X-ray angiograms. Phys Med Biol 2008;53:3807–20.

23. Chen S, Carroll J. 3D reconstruction of coronary arterial tree to optimize angiographic visualization. IEEE Trans Med Imaging 2000;19(4): 318–36.

24. Wink O, Kemkers R, Chen S, et al. Intra-procedural coronary intervention planning using hybrid 3-dimensional reconstruction techniques. Acad Radiol 2003;10:1433–41.

Enhanced X-Ray Visualization of Coronary Stents: Clinical Aspects

R. Kevin Rogers, MD, Andrew D. Michaels, MD, MAS, FACC, FAHA*

KEYWORDS

- StentBoost • Fluoroscopy
- Coronary artery disease
- Percutaneous coronary intervention • Stent

Percutaneous coronary intervention is a cornerstone in treating acute coronary syndromes and symptomatic obstructive coronary artery disease.[1–3] When compared to coronary angioplasty alone, the implantation of intracoronary stents increases rates of immediate and long-term angiographic and clinical success.[1,4] The risk of in-stent restenosis has been significantly reduced with the advent of drug-eluting stents.[1,5,6] However, acute in-stent thrombosis, though rare, remains a life-threatening, complication of stenting.[5,6]

Coronary stent underexpansion is a major contributor to in-stent restenosis and acute in-stent thrombosis, even in the drug-eluting stent era.[7,8] The current gold standard for detection of stent underexpansion is intravascular ultrasound (IVUS).[9–12] When performed in addition to conventional angiography to evaluate adequacy of stent expansion, IVUS improves mechanical results and decreases rates of target lesion revascularization.[13–16] However, IVUS is limited by professional and technical expertise, cost, procedural time, and the need of additional training of staff in catheterization laboratories. Fractional flow reserve measurements allow functional assessment of coronary stenosis, but have not been shown to reliably predict stent underexpansion.[17]

Traditional fluoroscopic and cineangiographic acquisition of deployed stents provides insufficient imaging resolution to assess stent expansion. Stent design advances have led to thinner stent struts, limiting x-ray imaging of deployed stents. Motion-corrected x-ray stent visualization (MXS) is a significant advance in x-ray technique that allows assessment of stent expansion. StentBoost (Philips Healthcare, Andover, Massachusetts),[18–21] an advanced fluoroscopic imaging alternative to IVUS, is superior to conventional angiography alone for assessing stent expansion. This technique provides enhanced stent visualization by eliminating motion artifact without adding procedural time or cost to conventional angiography.[18–21] Another MXS imaging modality, IC Stent (Siemens Medical Solutions USA, Malvern, Pennsylvania) is currently available, but published clinical data are pending.

MOTION-CORRECTED X-RAY STENT VISUALIZATION TECHNIQUES
Acquiring a StentBoost Image

Immediately after stent deployment and deflation of the stent delivery balloon, cineacquisition of the stented segment is performed with the deflated stent-deployment balloon positioned within the expanded stent of interest. Forty-five frames are acquired without injecting contrast.[18–21] This series of images is automatically transferred to a workstation (Philips Healthcare). From either tableside controls or the workstation, a region of

Supplementary material for this article can be found in the online version at doi:10.1016/j.ccl.2009.03.005.

Division of Cardiology, University of Utah Health Sciences Center, 30 N 1900 E, Room 4A100, Salt Lake City, UT 84132-2401, USA

* Corresponding author.

E-mail address: andrew.michaels@hsc.utah.edu (A.D. Michaels).

Cardiol Clin 27 (2009) 467–475
doi:10.1016/j.ccl.2009.03.005
0733-8651/09/$ – see front matter

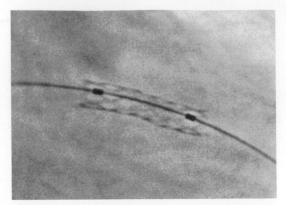

Fig. 1. Example of an MXS image. This image from the mid-left anterior descending coronary artery was obtained after postdilation with a noncompliant balloon 2 mm shorter than the stent.

interest is manually centered on the stent. Software corrects for motion by averaging images of the deployed stent from each cine frame in relation to the two balloon markers. The result, an enhanced image of the stent, is immediately viewable in the cardiac catheterization laboratory, with improved resolution and a superior signal-to-noise ratio that allows for identification of stent underexpansion (**Fig. 1**). To assess a change in stent expansion, MXS imaging may be repeated with a postdilatation balloon.

StentBoost Subtract

StentBoost Subtract is an advanced technique aimed at visualizing the stent in relation to the vessel lumen by using angiographic contrast injection.[19] In a manner similar to that for StentBoost acquisition, the deflated stent-deployment balloon for StentBoost Subtract remains positioned within

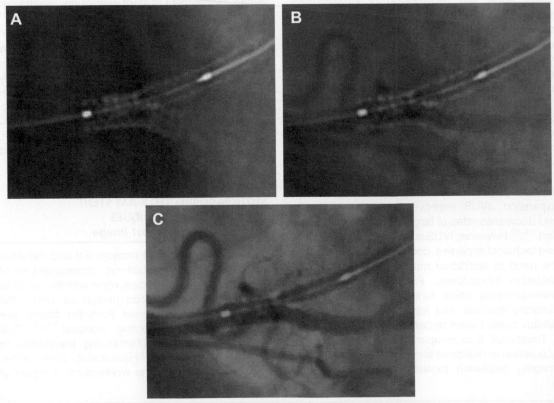

Fig. 2. This StentBoost Subtract movie (Video 1) shows the post-stenting angiographic and x-ray enhanced images of two stents in the distal right coronary artery covering both the posterior descending coronary artery and the posterolateral branch. (*A, B,* and *C*) Still frames from this video. (*A*) X-ray enhanced images of two stents before contrast injection. (*B*) Contrast visible within the vessel lumen as the stent image fades. Stent image completely faded; contrast visible within the vessel lumen. (*From* Garcia JA, Klein AJ, Wink O, et al. Use of Stent Boost Subtract for the precise evaluation of stent post PCI. Available at: www.tctmd.com. Accessed June 16, 2008; with permission.)

the deployed stent. Digital cineangiography is performed for 2 seconds without contrast injection and continued for 2 to 3 seconds while contrast is injected into the stented coronary segment. The series of images is automatically transferred to the workstation where motion-correction is performed as previously described (**Fig. 2** and Video 1 [Video 1 is available in the online version of this article at http://www.cardiology.theclinics.com/]).

Quantitative StentBoost Assessment

At the StentBoost workstation (but not at the tableside), image brightness can be adjusted. Individual angiographic frames can be excluded. In a method similar to that for quantitative angiography, the guiding catheter or the balloon markers provide a known distance for calibration. After calibration, the stent edges can be traced and measurements of the stent diameter at each point along the stent are available (**Fig. 3**).

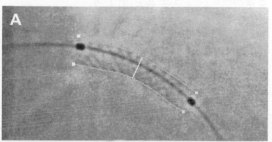

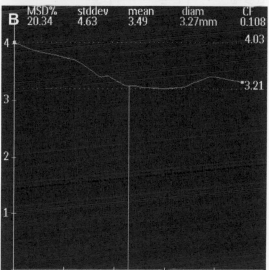

Fig. 3. Quantitative measurements of a deployed stent using MXS. (A) Enhanced x-ray image outlined. (B) Quantitative measurements of the stent diameter show distal tapering from 4.0 cm to 3.2 cm. MSD, minimal stenosis diameter percentage; stddev, standard deviation; diam, diameter; CF, calibration factor.

CLINICAL USE OF MOTION-CORRECTED X-RAY STENT VISUALIZATION TECHNIQUES

IVUS, the gold standard for evaluating adequate stent expansion, has been assessed in numerous clinical studies.[9–12] However, several factors limit more routine use of this modality. IVUS has been shown to increase procedural costs.[22–27] In the era of bare metal stents, this increase in procedural costs was offset by reduced rates of target lesion revascularization, resulting in no net cost increase. However, in the era of drug-eluting stents, restenosis rates have decreased, possibly diminishing the cost-effectiveness of IVUS. In addition to cost, a small risk of complications, particularly coronary spasm, is associated with the use of IVUS.[28]

The major limitation of qualitative and quantitative coronary angiography is decreased sensitivity in detecting stent underexpansion.[13] In fact, measurements of intracoronary stents by MXS appear to correlate more strongly with those of IVUS than do measurements by quantitative coronary angiography.[18] In a prospective, single-center study of 48 stents deployed in 30 patients, the correlation of minimum stent diameter between MXS and IVUS was higher ($r = 0.75$, $P < .0001$) compared to the correlation between quantitative coronary angiography and IVUS ($r = 0.65$, $P < .0001$).[18] In the Bland-Altman analysis, there was a smaller mean difference in minimum stent diameter between MXS and IVUS (0.043 mm) compared to the difference in minimum stent diameter between quantitative coronary angiography and IVUS (0.090 mm; $P < .001$). The MXS minimum diameter for detecting adequacy of stent expansion was 2.5 mm. This cutoff had a sensitivity of 88%, a specificity of 70%, a positive likelihood ratio of 2.9, and an area-under-the-curve c-statistic of 0.84 in diagnosing adequate stent expansion using IVUS as the gold standard. Limitations of this study included its small size, its single-center design, and the lack of blinding of investigators to measurements of the three imaging modalities.

MXS has several advantages compared to routine IVUS imaging of deployed stents (**Table 1**). Unlike IVUS, no additional equipment within the coronary artery is necessary to perform MXS, lowering the risk of mechanical complications. Second, MXS adds less than 1 minute of procedural time. Finally, MXS, which is virtually automated, requires less training of catheterization laboratory personnel. As for potential advantages of StentBoost Subtract, the technique enables additional assessment of malapposition and visualization of the stent in relation to angiographic

Table 1
Comparison of MXS, IVUS, and quantitative coronary angiography

	Correlation Coefficient with IVUS[a]	Cost	Advantages	Disadvantages
MXS	0.75	Initial capital costs include the StentBoost software and workstation; no per-patient costs	Little additional procedural time; no risk of mechanical complication; better correlation with IVUS compared to quantitative coronary angiography; better image resolution than cineangiography	Some training requirements for catheterization laboratory personnel; small amount of additional radiation; less useful in calcified segments; available from limited number of manufacturers
IVUS	—	Initial capital costs include the IVUS console; per-patient costs include the IVUS catheter and guide wire	Gold standard for stent underexpansion; useful for calcified lesions	Additional procedural time; increased risk of mechanical complications; more expensive than alternatives; requires additional training of catheterization laboratory personnel
Quantitative coronary angiography	0.65	Modest cost for quantitative coronary angiography software	Ease of use; least expensive; no additional radiation exposure if performed on routine post-stenting angiography	Least sensitive for stent underexpansion

[a] *Data from* Mishell JM, Vakharia KT, Ports TA, et al. Determination of adequate coronary stent expansion using StentBoost, a novel fluoroscopic image processing technique. Catheter Cardiovasc Interv 2007;69:84-93.

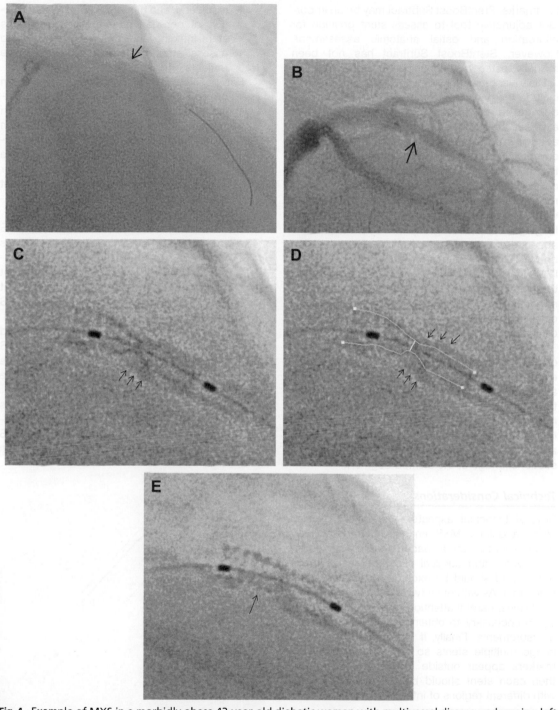

Fig. 4. Example of MXS in a morbidly obese 43-year-old diabetic woman with multivessel disease undergoing left anterior descending coronary artery stenting. Adequacy of stent expansion can be difficult to assess with conventional angiography in obese patients because of poor image quality with standard x-ray imaging after stent deployment. The arrow identifies the deployed stent on standard x-ray acquisition (*A*) and angiography (*B*). With the use of MXS (*C*), stent underexpansion becomes more evident, and extensive calcification under the stented segment can be appreciated (*arrows*). (*D*) The MXS stent border is traced; arrows show the areas of vessel calcification. (*E*) Improved but not perfect stent expansion on repeat MXS imaging postdilatation using a short noncompliant balloon (*arrow*).

landmarks. StentBoost Subtract may be an important adjunctive tool to assess stent position for bifurcation and ostial anatomic assessment. However, StentBoost Subtract has not been formally tested for these indications.

Disadvantages of MXS when compared to IVUS include the need for a slightly increased radiation dosage to the patient, which also potentially exposes the staff to more radiation. However, the acquisition of 45 frames with cineangiography is comparable to one angiographic run, which means that the additional radiation exposure is not clinically significant. Image resolution with MXS is reduced in heavily calcified vessels, a setting in which adequacy of stent expansion is challenging.[18] Michaels' group showed that, in the absence of coronary calcification, the correlation between the minimum stent diameter by MXS and IVUS was higher ($r = 0.99$, $P = .10$) compared to that seen in patients with presence of deep coronary calcium ($r = 0.84$, $P < .0001$) and superficial coronary calcium ($r = 0.57$, $P = .002$).[18] Finally, little clinical data or outcomes research exist for MXS.

MXS stent imaging, because it performed in only one projection, may under- or overestimate stent expansion, in comparison to IVUS imaging, which assesses the cross-sectional stent area. A potential future direction for these x-ray imaging techniques is to acquire rotational angiographic images with an MXS image processing system and then develop a three-dimensional cross-sectional image of the stented segment.[29]

Technical Considerations

Several technical aspects must be considered when acquiring MXS images. Fluoroscopically bright objects, such as pacemaker wires, sternotomy wires, and surgical clips, decrease image quality and should be excluded from the region of interest. As with other two-dimensional imaging modalities, careful attention to avoid foreshortening is necessary to obtain accurate images and measurements. Finally, if the operator wishes to image multiple stents so far apart that balloon markers appear outside the region of interest, then each stent should be imaged individually, with different regions of interest.

Potential Clinical Applications

Little has been reported in the literature on the clinical use of MXS. Below are clinical scenarios, based on several case studies and our experience, for which MXS may be useful:

For enhanced stent visualization in obese patients: Obesity decreases fluoroscopic

resolution, and hinders adequate visualization of coronary stents. MXS enhances stent imaging and improves the ability to assess stent underexpansion in obese patients (**Fig. 4**).

For positioning balloons and stents within previously stented segments: When posting a deployed stent, or positioning an overlapping additional stent, MXS can demonstrate the exact location of previously deployed stents. MXS may facilitate proper stent positioning in relation to prior stents. Additionally, the degree of stent overlap and stent expansion is easily assessed using MXS (**Fig. 5**).

As an alternative to IVUS: In some cases, MXS may provide a clinically effective, less expensive, and more time-efficient alternative to IVUS for assessing adequate stent deployment (**Fig. 6**). In other cases, it may not be possible to advance an IVUS catheter past the stent of interest (**Fig. 7**). If a balloon catheter can be advanced across a stenosed stent, then MXS imaging can be performed to assess expansion of the stenosed stent, and guide revascularization options.

For addressing bifurcation lesions: IVUS is especially cumbersome in cases of bifurcation lesions, where advancing the IVUS catheter across both vessel arms is

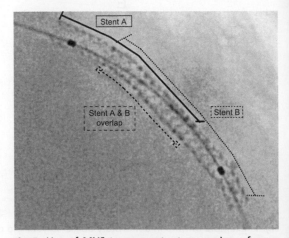

Fig. 5. Use of MXS to assess stent expansion of overlapping stents in the left anterior descending coronary artery. This patient presented with both bare-metal in-stent restenosis of stent A and severe native vessel stenoses distal to the stent. The patient underwent successful drug-eluting stenting (stent B) to cover both the in-stent restenotic and de novo lesions distal to the first stent. Both stents and the area of stent overlap are identified.

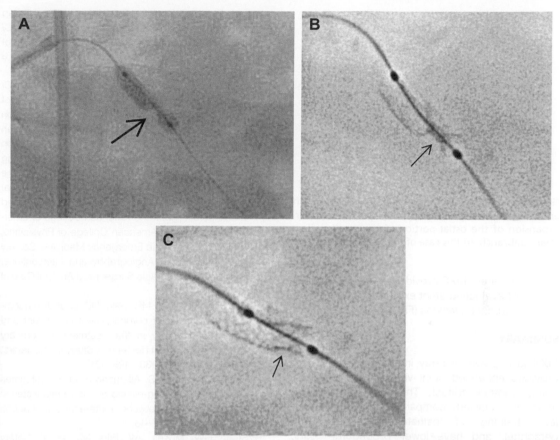

Fig. 6. Use of MXS as an alternative to IVUS. The patient is a morbidly obese 42-year-old man treated for acute thrombotic occlusion of the proximal left circumflex coronary artery after a ventricular fibrillation arrest. During predilation with a compliant balloon, it was difficult to appreciate whether the balloon was inflated fully, given the patient's obesity. (*A*) Angiography demonstrates severe underexpansion (*arrow*) during stent deployment at 18 atm. (*B*) The stent is clearly underexpanded (*arrow*) in resistant atherosclerotic lesion. (*C*) Stent expansion improved (*arrow*) after further balloon postdilatation.

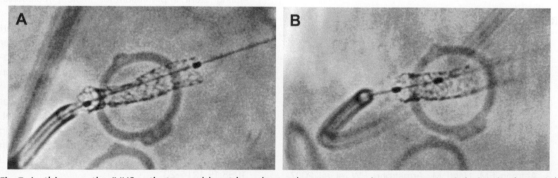

Fig. 7. In this case, the IVUS catheter could not be advanced past a severe in-stent restenotic lesion in the ostial portion of a saphenous vein graft. MXS was used to assess stent expansion. (*A*) The ostial portion of the stent was severely underexpanded by MXS imaging. (*B*) Improved stent expansion after further balloon postdilatation, This case also highlights the ability to use MXS in lesions close to radiopaque objects, such as a bypass graft marker.

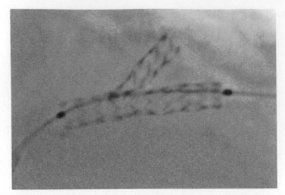

Fig. 8. MXS shows adequate expansion of the left anterior descending coronary artery stent, but under-expansion of the ostial portion of the smaller diagonal sidebranch, in this case of bifurcation T-stenting.

required. MXS provides an efficient means of evaluating stent expansion of stents for bifurcation lesions (**Fig. 8**).

SUMMARY

MXS is a powerful x-ray imaging modality that provides enhanced stent visualization by eliminating motion artifact. These techniques are more time-efficient compared to IVUS, require less training of catheterization laboratory personnel, and have lower procedural costs. However, scant clinical or outcome data are available for these x-ray imaging techniques. Though IVUS remains the gold standard for evaluation of the adequacy of stent expansion, MXS may be a viable adjunctive imaging tool in certain clinical scenarios.

APPENDIX: SUPPLEMENTARY MATERIAL

Supplementary material can be found, in the online version, at doi:10.1016/j.ccl.2009.03.005.

REFERENCES

1. King SB III, Smith SC Jr, Hirshfeld JW Jr, et al. 2007 focused update of the ACC/AHA/SCAI 2005 guideline update for percutaneous coronary intervention: a report of the American College of Cardiology/American Heart Association Task Force on Practice Guidelines: (2007 Writing Group to Review New Evidence and Update the 2005 ACC/AHA/SCAI Guideline Update for Percutaneous Coronary Intervention). J Am Coll Cardiol 2008;51:172–209.
2. Antman EM, Hand M, Armstrong PW, et al. 2007 focused update of the ACC/AHA 2004 guidelines for the management of patients with ST-elevation myocardial infarction: a report of the American College of Cardiology/American Heart Association Task Force on Practice Guidelines (Writing Group to Review New Evidence and Update the ACC/AHA 2004 Guidelines for the Management of Patients With ST-Elevation Myocardial Infarction). J Am Coll Cardiol 2008;51:210–47.
3. Anderson JL, Adams CD, Antman EM, et al. ACC/AHA 2007 guidelines for the management of patients with unstable angina/non–ST-elevation myocardial infarction: a report of the American College of Cardiology/American Heart Association Task Force on Practice Guidelines (Writing Committee to Revise the 2002 Guidelines for the Management of Patients With Unstable Angina/Non–ST-Elevation Myocardial Infarction): developed in collaboration with the American College of Emergency Physicians, American College of Physicians, Society for Academic Emergency Medicine, Society for Cardiovascular Angiography and Interventions, and Society of Thoracic Surgeons. J Am Coll Cardiol 2007;50:e1–157.
4. Fischman DL, Leon MB, Baim DS, et al. A randomized comparison of coronary-stent placement and balloon angioplasty in the treatment of coronary artery disease. Stent Restenosis Study Investigators. N Engl J Med 1994;331:496–501.
5. Stettler C, Wandel S, Allemann S, et al. Outcomes associated with drug-eluting and bare-metal stents: a collaborative network meta-analysis. Lancet. 2007;370(9591):937–48.
6. Stone GW, Moses JW, Ellis SG, et al. Safety and efficacy of sirolimus- and paclitaxel-eluting coronary stents. N Engl J Med. 2007;356(10):998–1008.
7. Fujii K, Carlier SG, Mintz GS, et al. Stent underexpansion and residual reference segment stenosis are related to stent thrombosis after sirolimus-eluting stent implantation: an intravascular ultrasound study. J Am Coll Cardiol 2005;45:995–8.
8. Fujii K, Mintz GS, Kobayashi Y, et al. Contribution of stent underexpansion to recurrence after sirolimus-eluting stent implantation for in-stent restenosis. Circulation 2004;109:1085–8.
9. de Feyter PJ, Kay P, Disco C, et al. Reference chart derived from post-stent-implantation intravascular ultrasound predictors of 6-month expected restenosis on quantitative coronary angiography. Circulation 1999;100:1777–83.
10. de Jaegere P, Mudra H, Figulla H, et al. Intravascular ultrasound-guided optimized stent deployment. Immediate and 6 months clinical and angiographic results from the Multicenter Ultrasound Stenting in Coronaries Study (MUSIC Study). Eur Heart J 1998;19:1214–23.
11. Hoffmann R, Mintz GS, Mehran R, et al. Intravascular ultrasound predictors of angiographic restenosis in lesions treated with Palmaz-Schatz stents. J Am Coll Cardiol 1998;31:43–9.

12. Mintz GS, Nissen SE, Anderson WD, et al. ACC clinical expert consensus document on standards for the acquisition, measurement and reporting of intravascular ultrasound studies: a report of the American College of Cardiology Task Force on Clinical Expert Consensus Documents (Committee to Develop a Clinical Expert Consensus Document on Standards for Acquisition, Measurement and Reporting of Intravascular Ultrasound Studies [IVUS]). J Am Coll Cardiol 2001;37:1478–92.

13. Blasini R, Neumann FJ, Schmitt C, et al. Comparison of angiography and intravascular ultrasound for the assessment of lumen size after coronary stent placement: impact of dilation pressures. Cathet Cardiovasc Diagn 1997;42:113–9.

14. Colombo A, Hall P, Nakamura S, et al. Intracoronary stenting without anticoagulation accomplished with intravascular ultrasound guidance. Circulation 1995;91:1676–88.

15. Goldberg SL, Colombo A, Nakamura S, et al. Benefit of intracoronary ultrasound in the deployment of Palmaz-Schatz stents. J Am Coll Cardiol 1994;24:996–1003.

16. Fitzgerald PJ, Oshima A, Hayase M, et al. Final results of the Can Routine Ultrasound Influence Stent Expansion (CRUISE) study. Circulation 2000;102:523–30.

17. Fearon WF, Luna J, Samady H, et al. Fractional flow reserve compared with intravascular ultrasound guidance for optimizing stent deployment. Circulation 2001;104:1917–22.

18. Mishell JM, Vakharia KT, Ports TA, et al. Determination of adequate coronary stent expansion using StentBoost, a novel fluoroscopic image processing technique. Catheter Cardiovasc Interv 2007;69:84–93.

19. Agostoni P, Verheye S. Bifurcation stenting with a dedicated biolimus-eluting stent: X-ray visual enhancement of the final angiographic result with "StentBoost Subtract". Catheter Cardiovasc Interv 2007;70:233–6.

20. Agostoni P, Verheye S, Vermeersch P, et al. "Virtual" in-vivo bench test for bifurcation stenting with "Stent-Boost." Int J Cardiol 2008;133:67–9.

21. Vydt T, Van Langenhove G. Facilitated recognition of an undeployed stent with StentBoost. Int J Cardiol 2006;112:397–8.

22. Berry E, Kelly S, Hutton J, et al. Intravascular ultrasound-guided interventions in coronary artery disease: a systematic literature review, with decision-analytic modelling, of outcomes and cost-effectiveness. Health Technol Assess 2000;4:1–117.

23. Choi JW, Goodreau LM, Davidson CJ. Resource utilization and clinical outcomes of coronary stenting: a comparison of intravascular ultrasound and angiographical guided stent implantation. Am Heart J 2001;142:112–8.

24. Gaster AL, Slothuus Skjoldborg U, Larsen J, et al. Continued improvement of clinical outcome and cost effectiveness following intravascular ultrasound guided PCI: insights from a prospective, randomised study. Heart 2003;89:1043–9.

25. Gaster AL, Slothuus U, Larsen J, et al. Cost-effectiveness analysis of intravascular ultrasound guided percutaneous coronary intervention versus conventional percutaneous coronary intervention. Scand Cardiovasc J 2001;35:80–5.

26. Mueller C, Hodgson JM, Schindler C, et al. Cost-effectiveness of intracoronary ultrasound for percutaneous coronary interventions. Am J Cardiol 2003;91:143–7.

27. Schiele F, Meneveau N, Seronde MF, et al. Medical costs of intravascular ultrasound optimization of stent deployment. Results of the multicenter randomized 'REStenosis after Intravascular ultrasound STenting' (RESIST) study. Int J Cardiovasc Intervent 2000;3:207–13.

28. Hausmann D, Erbel R, Alibelli-Chemarin MJ, et al. The safety of intracoronary ultrasound. A multicenter survey of 2207 examinations. Circulation 1995;91:623–30.

29. Schaefer D, Movassaghi B, Grass M, et al. Three-dimensional reconstruction of coronary stents in vivo based on motion compensated X-ray angiography. Med Image Comput Assist Interv 2006;9:177–84.

Advanced Visibility Enhancement for Stents and Other Devices: Image Processing Aspects

Gert Schoonenberg, MSc[a,b,*], Raoul Florent, MSc[c]

KEYWORDS

- Percutaneous coronary intervention
- Coronary artery disease • Image enhancement
- Device reconstruction • Implantable cardiovascular devices

Cardiac devices, such as stents, are being implanted daily worldwide. To ensure the proper outcome of these procedures, clinicians must be able to see how these devices are deployed. Reports have noted inadequate deployment of stents, leading to incomplete apposition to the vessel wall.[1,2] Late thrombosis and in-stent restenosis also can occur. It is therefore important that the deployment of devices can be analyzed at the time of deployment and immediately improved if necessary.

Visualization of these deployed stents is especially important now, in the era of the newer drug-eluting stents because they are less radiopaque than bare metal stents and therefore more difficult to see with conventional x-ray coronary angiography. To evaluate full stent deployment, interventionalists sometimes make use of intravascular ultrasound (IVUS), although this practice remains relatively limited in most countries. An interesting alternative consists in relying on enhanced stent visualization tools for x-ray sequences, such as StentBoost (Philips Healthcare, Best, The Netherlands), IC Stent (Siemens Healthcare, Erlangen, Germany), or StentOptimizer (Paieon Inc., New York, New York). These latter tools enable the visualization and analysis of a deployed stent in one projection direction.

Three-dimensional (3D) stent reconstruction has been developed to allow enhanced stent visualization and measurements in three instead of two dimensions. All those visibility-enhancement techniques using x-ray–based devices rely on unique features in the acquired images to allow for motion compensation of the object of interest, which, together with temporal integration or reconstruction, forms the basis of device visualization enhancement. This article gives an overview of the different methods used for enhanced stent visualization, describes the studies evaluating these methods, and summarizes results of these methods on other cardiac and noncardiac devices.

STENT-VISIBILITY ENHANCEMENT

The general method for improving visibility of stents during percutaneous coronary intervention involves the creation of an enhanced exposure image that clearly outlines the geometry of the deployed stent from a fixed viewing direction. The enhancement is achieved by employing a motion-compensation process and temporal integration of the image sequence to increase contrast visibility.

a Department of Cardiovascular Innovation, Business Unit Cardio/Vascular X-Ray, Philips Healthcare, Veenpluis 4-6, 5680 DA Best, The Netherlands.
b Division Biomedical Imaging and Modeling, Department of Biomedical Engineering, Eindhoven University of Technology, Den Dolech 2, 5600 MB Eindhoven, The Netherlands
c Medisys Research Lab, Philips Healthcare, 33 rue de Verdun, 92156 Suresnes Cedex, France
* Corresponding author.
E-mail address: gert.schoonenberg@philips.com (G. Schoonenberg).

Cardiol Clin 27 (2009) 477–490
doi:10.1016/j.ccl.2009.03.007

Processing Steps

The motion-compensation process identifies the stent region in each projection image to register the series of sequential images. This can be done in various ways. One of the common methods reported in the literature is the landmark-based technique to identify the stent region.[3–9] Those methods typically use balloon markers for identification of the stent region. An extension to this approach uses, in addition to the balloon markers, the wire between the balloon markers.[10] Of course, approaches based on markers and wires can only be effective if the balloon delivery system remains in place immediately after stent deployment. Also, one could argue that, once deployed, the stent might move somewhat independently of the deployment setup, which makes balloon catheter–based registration suboptimal. To circumvent those issues, one approach based on deformable boundary detection[11] has been proposed to localize the stent by detection of the outer contour of the stent in the projection images. Another technique based on a layer decomposition algorithm has been proposed. With this technique, the series of cine images is decomposed into different moving layers.[12] As a result of this decomposition, the stent is shown in one layer while background structures are contained in other layers. These methods all require, as a first step, the application of a segmentation process for identification of landmarks (eg, balloon markers, the wire, or the stent contour) to accurately localize the stent region. In the next step, these landmarks need to be registered throughout the image sequence to compensate for combined cardiac and respiratory motion. When only the markers are used as landmarks, an affine transformation for each frame, consisting of translation, rotation, and stretching in two dimensions, suffices for the registration process (**Fig. 1**). If the curved wire or the contour of the stent is used as the landmark, an elastic transformation will be needed to take into account nonlinear movement (ie, stent bending) of the object throughout the cardiac cycle and allow for more accurate registration. In the remainder of this article, the affine transformation for 2D motion compensation is assumed. However, more advanced transformations can be used as well.

With the completion of the registration process, the transformed image is displayed and clinicians may adjust contrast and brightness to obtain the best view of the stent. Additionally, other typical image processing techniques can be applied, such as zoom-in on region of interest (ROI), adaptation of the gray-level dynamics to the selected stent-centric ROI, histogram manipulation in selective regions, and edge enhancement. As a result, the spatial processing methods in conjunction with the temporal integration process enable a much clearer and more useful view of the stent. The detailed steps in the process of enhancing the image of the stent are summarized in **Fig. 2**. Various cases are shown in **Fig. 3** to demonstrate the effectiveness and usefulness of the process for enhanced stent visualization based on StentBoost software.

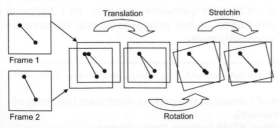

Fig. 1. Registration of two frames from the exposure sequence (Frame 1 and Frame 2) using an affine transformation consisting of translation, rotation, and stretching.

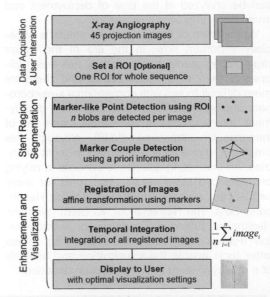

Fig. 2. Processing steps for enhancing stents in x-ray exposure sequences: acquiring projection images; setting an optional region of interest (ROI); marker-couple detection based on marker detection; boosting of the image by registering all frames using an affine transformation and temporal integration of these registered images; and finally displaying the end result to the user with optimal visualization settings.

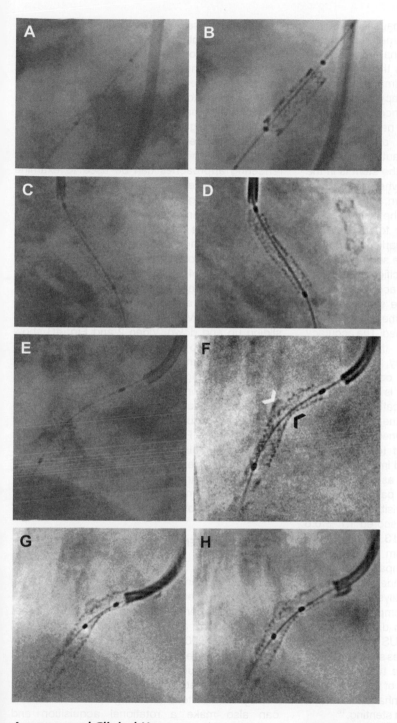

Fig. 3. Various StentBoost cases. (*A*) An image from an exposure sequence with a stent and (*B*) the corresponding enhanced stent image. (*C*) An image from an exposure sequence with a longer and more curved stent and (*D*) the corresponding enhanced stent image. (*E–H*) Various images from a stent deployment where calcifications where present. (*E*) Image from an exposure sequence with a deployed 3.5 × 20-mm Taxus stent (Boston Scientific, Maple Grove, Minnesota) dilated at 14 atm. (*F*) An enhanced stent image showing a calcification (*white arrow*) and stent underdeployment (*black arrow*). (*G*) Positioning of a noncompliant 10/ 4.0-mm Extensor balloon (Medronic, Santa Rosa, California) dilated at 22 atm. (*H*) Result shows improved stent expansion.

Accuracy and Clinical Use

Although stent visibility has been greatly improved in the enhanced images, the process of obtaining accurate and quantitative estimates of the stent's geometry after it has been implanted (eg, 3D length and diameters) is tricky. This is because the projection image is not useful for recovering 3D morphology and the relative position (ie, the location and orientation) of an object (eg, the implanted stent) with respect to the imaging system. Additionally, because of the characteristics of cone-beam imaging projection, an object farther away from the detector will appear bigger in the projection image than an object near the detector. Therefore a calibration process is still needed to perform any traditional 2D quantitative measurements based on the enhanced images. Calibration is a burden to the operator because it requires manual selection of a calibration method and, depending on the method, additional user interaction. Calibration is not needed in the workflow of generating the enhanced stent images, but it is necessary to validate the accuracy of this technique. The pixel size of the enhanced images can be calibrated in different ways, namely catheter calibration, marker calibration, and automatic pixel-based calibration. The automatic pixel-based calibration assumes that the stent is in the isocenter of the C-arm systems, where the calibration factor (mm/pixel) is known, because the distance from the generator to the isocenter and the distance from the isocenter to the detector are known. With catheter and marker calibration, a catheter or marker needs to be segmented and their dimensions need to be specified to calculate the calibration factor. To get an accurate calibration, the catheter must be in the same plane as the stent (in a plane parallel to the detector) and the stent must not be foreshortened. The accuracy can fluctuate depending on the calibration method, segmentation accuracy, and operator skills. Measurement errors can occur when the stent is foreshortened, the stent is not in the isocenter of the system, and the catheter used for calibration is not in the same plane.

Various studies have examined the clinical usefulness of this enhancement technique. The stent visibility of those enhanced images is better than that of the standard images, as demonstrated in a study of 27 consecutive patients and 35 stents.[3,13] On a scale from 1 (not visible) to 5 (crystal clear), the conventional images scored 1.7 ± 0.6 and the enhanced images scored 3.5 ± 0.8. Quantitative stent measurements from the enhanced images and IVUS were compared in three studies.[3,14,15] One study also made a comparison with quantitative coronary analysis (**Table 1**). Various measurements where compared between StentBoost and IVUS: minimum diameter, mean diameter, and area ratios for IVUS with diameter ratios for 2D StentBoost. All studies show a medium to large correlation between the two modalities. Besides accuracy and validation of this technique, the clinical use of stent visibility enhancement tools has been reported for bifurcation stenting.[16]

STENTBOOST SUBTRACT

An extension to the aforementioned enhanced angiograms is a tool called StentBoost Subtract (Philips Healthcare, Best, The Netherlands). By showing the stent in relation to the vessel wall, this tool, in addition to enhancing stent visibility, enables operators to assess the apposition of the stent to the vessel wall. This is achieved by modifying the protocol as originally used for StentBoost image acquisition. Contrast agent is injected halfway during the acquisition so that the coronary segment of interest is opacified and included in the subsequently acquired image sequence. The frames with the same cardiac phase (eg, end diastole) in the images of coronary arterial segment and the enhanced StentBoost images are identified so that they can be combined. Various rendering approaches can be used to examine these two images. The simplest approach is to display the images side by side. However, with this approach, interpreting the relation between the stent and the vessel wall is still difficult. Therefore, dynamic approaches were evaluated that combine the two images in movie loops. Videos 1 to 4 and **Fig. 4** show four different approaches of these animations (videos available in the online version of this article at http://www.cardiology. theclinics.com). Video 1 and **Fig. 4**A show a curtain sliding up and down. Video 2 and **Fig. 4**B show blinds sliding to the left. Video 3 and **Fig. 4**C show a fade-in and fade-out of the enhanced stent image on the angiogram image. Video 4 and **Fig. 4**D show results in the similar way with a gray-scale inverted enhanced stent image. This latter visualization method became the default visualization method for the Philips StentBoost Subtract tool. Clinical use of this tool has typically been reported in bifurcation stenting cases.[16–18] An example of StentBoost Subtract in bifurcation stenting is illustrated in five frames from the fade-in and fade-out animation as shown in **Fig. 5**.

STENT ENHANCEMENT USING ROTATIONAL ACQUISITION

Stent visibility enhancement is often done using two viewing directions.[3] If the stent is underdeployed in a certain viewing direction, another exposure from a viewing direction rotated by approximately 90° around the axis of the stent is needed to correctly visualize this underdeployment. A minimum of two viewing directions is therefore needed to adequately evaluate stent deployment. Instead of setting up two views, one can also make a rotational acquisition and enhance this run. An apparent problem is the changing projected shape of the device throughout the run, which makes automatic detection of the stent region and registration more difficult. Automated marker-based segmentation of the stent region is feasible for rotational acquisitions.[9] The enhancement of rotational runs is possible, but due to changing geometry between successive images only a limited number of

Table 1
Validation studies of StentBoost

Study	Hanekamp, Koolen, et al[3,13]	Conway et al[14]		Mishell et al[15]	
Number of patients	27	33		30	
Number of coronary stents	35	43		48	
Gold standard	IVUS	IVUS		IVUS	QCA
Measurement	Mean diameter for IVUS and StentBoost	Ratio minimum/mean stent cross-sectional area for IVUS and ratio minimum/mean diameter for StentBoost	Ratio minimum/maximum stent cross-sectional area for IVUS and ratio minimum/maximum diameter for StentBoost	Minimum diameter for IVUS and StentBoost	Minimum diameter for QCA and StentBoost
Correlation coefficient method	—	Two-tailed Spearman	Two-tailed Spearman	Pearson product-moment	Pearson product-moment
Correlation coefficient	0.819 ± 0.122	0.44	0.57	0.75	0.49
P value	<.05	.003	<.001	<.0001	.0004

Abbreviation: QCA, quantitative coronary analysis.

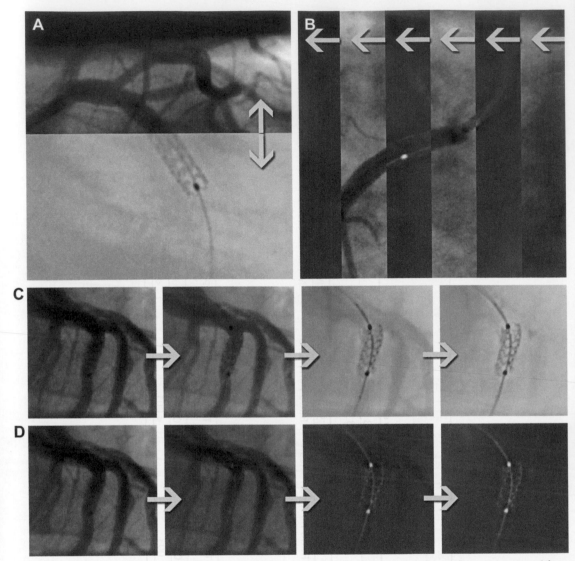

Fig. 4. Overview of different animated visualization modes for displaying an enhanced stent image with an angiogram. (*A*) One frame of curtain sliding up and down. (*B*) One frame of blinds sliding to the left. (*C*) four frames of fade-in and fade-out animation. (*D*) Four frames of fade-in and fade-out animation, with grayscale-inverted enhanced stent image. See also corresponding Movies 1 through 4.

frames can be integrated for each individual enhanced image.[19] Because using more frames in the enhancement phase theoretically results in better images, this limitation on the number of frames could be a shortcoming. A rotational acquisition over 90° will obtain similar information as two fixed-view acquisitions at a similar dose. **Fig. 6** shows an enhanced image from a rotational acquisition of a coronary stent.

THREE-DIMENSIONAL STENT RECONSTRUCTION

3D motion-compensated volumetric stent reconstruction has been developed to give insight into the 3D geometry of the deployed stent. These

projection images, instead of being used to enhance the image of the stent, are used to reconstruct the stent in a volumetric dataset. In principle, the exposure images can be motion-compensated in the same way as previously shown in **Fig. 1** for 2D stent-visualization enhancement. After motion compensation, a standard cone-beam–based reconstruction method can be used to generate the volumetric dataset. Phantom and animal studies have indeed shown that stents can be reconstructed this way assuming that the motion of the markers on the balloon catheter is equal to the motion of the stent.[6,20] Pilot studies of 3D stent reconstruction in humans using an image intensifier system[21,22] and a flat panel detector[23] have shown the feasibility of

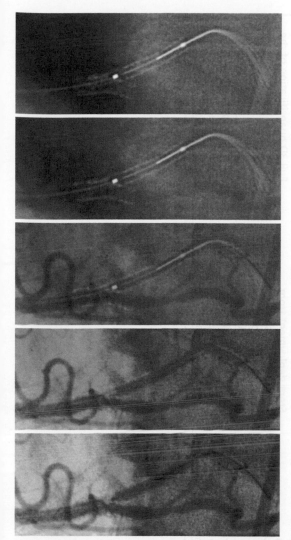

Fig. 5. StentBoost Subtract (Philips Healthcare, Best, The Netherlands) in a bifurcation stenting case. (*Top* to *bottom*) Five images from a fade-in, fade-out sequence of the enhanced stent image and an angiogram.

this technology in a clinical setting. A recent publication[9] shows that the whole process of 3D stent reconstruction can be automated. However, 3D stent reconstruction is clinically and technically more challenging than enhancing 2D projection images. **Table 2** shows an overview of these enhancement and reconstruction techniques and summarizes some key elements. The following section describes in more detail the clinical workflow, the image processing steps, and clinical tools for 3D stent reconstruction.

Clinical Workflow and Data Processing

A rotational acquisition starts with isocentering the device in the C-arm system to ensure that the device will be visible throughout the acquisition. Typically, patients are instructed to hold their breath during the rotational run to minimize respiratory motion. A calibrated monoplane C-arm system will then rotate 180°, generating exposure images at 30 Hz for a duration of 5 to 7 seconds.[6,9] The estimated effective dose for a typical acquisition of 7 seconds at 30 Hz using a torso phantom (posterior-anterior diameter 24 cm, left-right diameter 30 cm) is 0.7 millisievert (mSv) based on an estimated dose area product with an effective dose conversion factor of $0.183 \text{ mSv/(Gy} \times \text{cm}^2)$.[24] After the acquisition, the projection images are available for review and the processing of the data can start.

Schoonenberg and colleagues[9] report fully automatic processing in 9 out of 10 coronary stents in humans. **Fig. 7** gives an overview of this fully automatic process. First the operator can set an optional ROI to indicate the stent region and thus reduce the search space for the subsequent automated processing steps. The stent regions are automatically identified in each projection image. The only a priori information

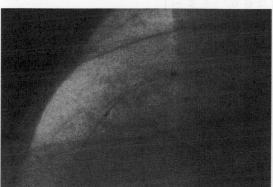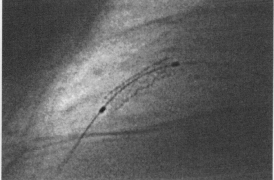

Fig. 6. Application of StentBoost in a rotational run. (*Left*) Single unenhanced image of the Taxus Express[2] 3.0 × 16-mm stent (Boston Scientific, Maple Grove, Minnesota) of the rotational acquisition. (*Right*) Enhanced image of this stent placed in the left anterior descending artery.

Table 2
Overview of 2D and 3D device enhancement techniques

	2D Device Enhancement	2D Rotational Device Enhancement	3D Device Enhancement
Commercially available	Yes	No	No
Acquisition	Static viewing direction	Short rotation: 90°	Long rotation: 180°
Projection images	45	90	157–211
Advantages	Very fast processing (order of magnitude seconds)	Stent deployment from various angles using dose similar to that for 2 static-view acquisitions	Full 3D quantification of the stent
Disadvantages	Enhanced images from 1 viewing direction at a time; only measurements in 2D	Rotational acquisition limits enhancement; only measurements in 2D	Dose; Slow processing (order of magnitude minutes)

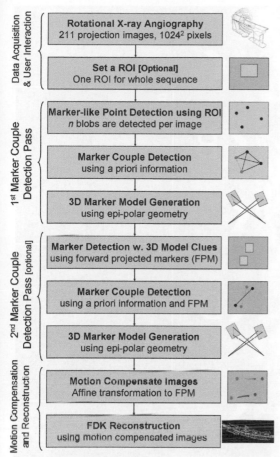

Fig. 7. Processing steps of 3D stent reconstruction. ROI, region of interest.

for detecting the stent region is the need to identify two periodically moving markers in each projection image. Due to foreshortening, the distance between these markers can vary in the projection images. Also, due to the rotation of the C-arm system, the orientation of these projected markers can vary. First the algorithm tries to find as many markerlike structures as possible and then it tries to select the best marker couple for each frame. The marker couple then defines the stent region in an image. Because images are acquired at high frame speed (30 Hz), small angular difference between frames (less than 1°), and relative low heart rate (approximately 1 Hz), the displacement of the markers between successive frames of the rotational run is limited. This temporal constraint helps the algorithm finding the correct solution throughout the acquisition. The typical percentage of correct marker-couple detection (true positives) in the images of a rotational acquisition is about 42% without a ROI and 79% with a ROI with respectively 15% and 5% false-positive detections.[9]

To improve these results, a second marker-couple detection step is introduced. This uses a 3D model of the markers generated from the first step. Two frames with the highest likelihood of correct marker-couple detection are used to model the two markers in 3D using epi-polar geometry. By forward-projecting the 3D model of markers on the acquired image, a location in the projection image is calculated. This location serves to determine an ROI for an additional stent region detection step. The steps of markerlike point detection, marker-couple selection, and 3D marker model generation are repeated to improve the results (see optional second marker-couple detection pass in **Fig. 7**).

The 3D model of markers generated from the second step is used as the reference state to which the projection images will be motion-compensated. The 3D model is forward-projected on the acquired image and the difference between the forward-projected markers and the detected markers is a measure of the motion of the stent. By warping the images from the detected positions to the forward-projected reference position, the motion can be corrected (see **Fig. 1**). A standard cone-beam reconstruction method can be applied to the motion-compensated images, resulting in a motion-compensated reconstruction of the stent.

Visualization Tool

The 3D reconstructed volume can be displayed with standard visualization techniques, such as volume rendering. The operator can freely zoom, pan, and rotate the reconstructed stent. Additionally, the stent reconstruction can also be used in a more tailored visualization technique called *virtual pullback*. This unique tool allows an automatic moving cut plane perpendicular to the guide wire to move and generate planar reformats similar to those obtained with IVUS. **Fig. 8** shows a volume-rendered reconstructed stent and five automatically generated cross-sectional images. Both the 3D volume-rendered reconstructed stent and the automatically generated cross-sectional images can be used for taking measurements.

Accuracy

Because a calibrated C-arm system was used to generate the data, measurements are assumed to be highly accurate. Preliminary and unpublished results on comparing the 3D stent reconstructions and cross-section images with IVUS in one patient show a strong correlation of minimal and maximum diameter and cross-sectional area measurements between the two modalities. Two

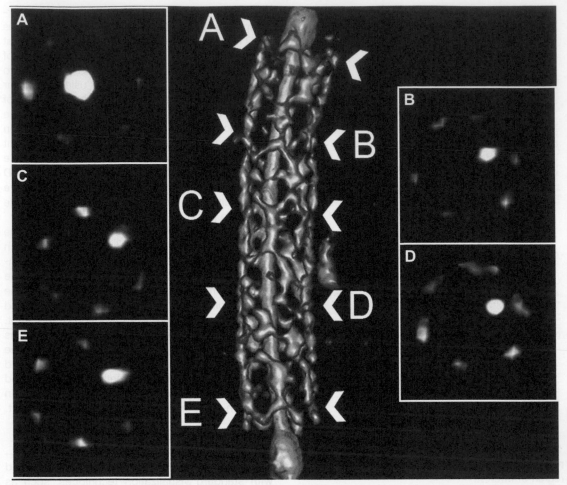

Fig. 8. Volume-rendered reconstructed Taxus Express[2] 3.0 × 16-mm stent (Boston Scientific, Maple Grove, Minnesota) with five cross-sectional views (virtual pullback). Arrows indicate how views A through E correspond to locations. In image A, thick structure in the middle is the marker on the balloon wire. In images B through E, the wire is visible. The other dots in images A through E are stent struts. The cross sections of the stent are circular and no underexpansion is observed.

human observers manually segmented the stent contour in the IVUS images and in the cross-sectional images generated from the 3D reconstructed stent. Based on these contours, cross-sectional stent area, minimum stent diameter, and maximum stent diameter are calculated. **Fig. 9** shows an IVUS frame (A) and the segmented stent contour (B) and a cross-sectional view of the x-ray–based reconstruction (C) and the segmented stent contour (D). X-ray–based 3D stent reconstruction overestimates the measured values compared with IVUS by 1% to 5% in this single-case comparison. In both modalities, the diameter and surface area values are smaller in the more distal part as expected from physiologic vessel tapering.

RESULTS OF ENHANCEMENT OF OTHER CARDIOVASCULAR DEVICES

The techniques of 2D stent enhancement, 2D rotational stent enhancement, and 3D stent reconstruction can also be applied to other devices that have markers or markerlike features. **Table 2** shows an overview of these device enhancement techniques and summarizes some key elements. These techniques can of course be applied to cardiac devices that exhibit cyclic motion, but they are also potentially beneficial for other noncardiac vascular devices. We will show the results of these techniques applied to two other devices in cardiac and noncardiac applications. First an atrial septal defect closure device is imaged using the rotational acquisition protocol.

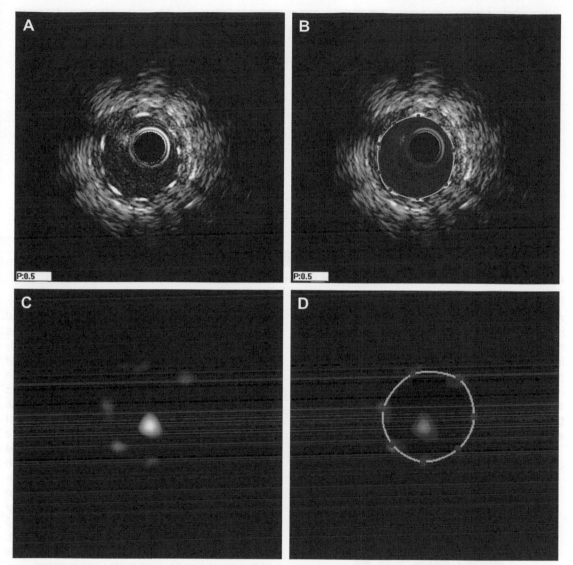

Fig. 9. Segmentation results of one IVUS frame and one cross-section image of the reconstructed stent. (*A*) IVUS image. (*B*) Corresponding stent segmentation. (*C*) Cross-sectional image of the reconstructed stent. (*D*) Corresponding stent segmentation.

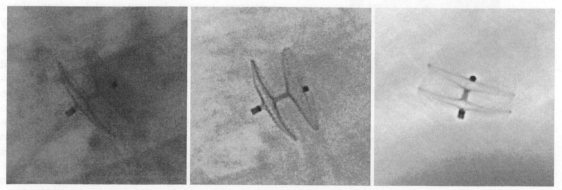

Fig. 10. (*Left*) Exposure image from a rotational acquisition of an atrial septal defect closure device. (*Middle*) Corresponding enhanced stent image. (*Right*) Enhanced image from a different viewing direction.

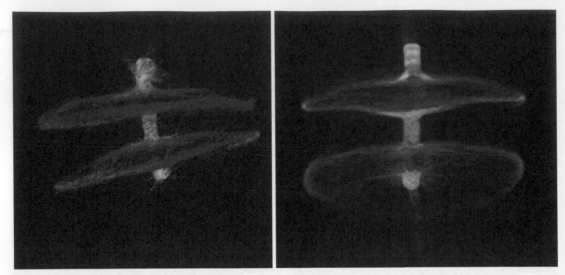

Fig. 11. Two motion-compensated reconstructions of closure devices.

Atrial septal defect closure devices typically do not have markers. However, their wire frame, made of Nitinol, an alloy of nickel and titanium, features two inherent markerlike parts: the two connection points of all wires. These markerlike parts are automatically identified throughout the rotational run as if they were balloon markers. Rotational StentBoost and 3D stent reconstruction are then applied (**Figs. 10** and **11**).

A noncardiac 6.0 × 18-mm ParaMount Mini GPS (ev3 Inc., Plymouth, Minnesota) stent was placed after pre-dilation within the right renal artery ostium. Then a rotational acquisition was performed. This particular stent has four radiopaque tantalum markers built into each end of the stent. Our automated algorithm[9] was unable to coherently select the same two markers throughout the run. Manual interaction was needed to identify one marker on each end of the stent. After this manual step, all frames were motion-compensated automatically and the whole sequence was reconstructed. Even though motion in the renal artery is significantly less than in coronaries, it is enough to decrease image quality to unacceptable levels. **Fig. 12** shows the motion-compensated reconstructed stent. In Video 5 (available in the online version of this article at: http://www.cardiology.theclinics.com), the struts of this stent can be even better appreciated.

SUMMARY

A percutaneous intervention involving vascular devices cannot be successful unless those devices are precisely implanted and properly deployed. Traditionally stent expansion can be assessed using IVUS. Routine use of IVUS may result in improved stent expansion;[25] however, it is not routinely performed in all patients undergoing percutaneous interventions. Disadvantages of IVUS are extra cost, additional procedure time, and increased risk of mechanical complications. Other implanted vascular devices are also often imaged with different modalities, such as 3D transesophageal echocardiography and intracardiac echo to guide interventional procedures and verify proper device placement. Bringing other modalities to the catheterization laboratory

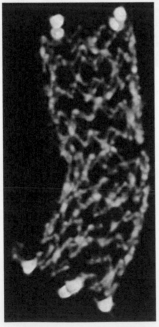

Fig. 12. Image of 3D reconstructed vascular stent using motion compensation. See also Movie 5.

typically lengthens the procedural time, especially when it is a mobile system, but also when it is integrated within the x-ray suite. It also requires additional capital investments and training of the catheterization laboratory staff.

Over the last decade, researchers have developed technology that enables better visualization and analysis tools based on the x-ray system itself. With the introduction of x-ray–based 2D stent enhancement tools, the visibility of the deployed stent has been improved in the exposure sequences.[3] This technique is an alternative to IVUS and commercially available from the main manufacturers of cardiovascular x-ray suite equipment. Disadvantages of this technique are a small additional amount of radiation. However, this technique requires less additional procedural time and no extra cost per patient, except for the initial costs of the software itself. A clear limitation of this technique remains the nature of 2D projection, which makes it impossible to generate cross-sectional images like those generated with IVUS. A way to tackle this problem is to make 3D reconstructions in a manner similar to that used in neurovascular imaging.

Fully automated, motion-compensated, 3D device reconstruction based on rotational x-ray angiography has been developed for cardiovascular implantable devices that exhibit motion. One apparent advantage of this angiography over the other x-ray–based 2D enhancement tools is that it offers the possibility of obtaining accurate measurements in 3D. However, this advantage has yet to be proven in a large-scale comparison study with IVUS. Device reconstruction does not provide any information regarding surrounding tissue during device implantation; it only has the potential to show calcifications. This is a shortcoming compared with IVUS.

Another limitation of the 3D motion-compensated reconstruction technology is foreshortening of the device in parts of the rotational run. This is reported for cardiac stents[9] and typically occurs in the proximal and distal portions of all coronary vessels. This limitation is clinically pertinent given the amount of myocardium at risk if a proximal stent were to have acute stent thrombosis. Hence, for stents in these locations, the operator should rely on 2D enhancement. In the future, this limitation might be addressed by changing the image-acquisition trajectory to reduce foreshortening of the device or by improved motion-compensation techniques.

A third limitation of this technique is that, because markers are required, it can only be performed during stent implantation and not during follow-up procedures. However, if in the future stents are provided with markers, or automated detection using the stent contour is possible in combination with motion compensation, this technique might be useful for follow-up procedures.

Because 3D device reconstruction is a low-risk, cost-effective, time-efficient method, it might become an alternative for 2D enhanced device visualization and the ultrasound-based modalities to verify proper device placement.

ACKNOWLEDGMENTS

The authors would like to acknowledge John Carroll, MD, and the Cardiac Catheterization Laboratory at the University of Colorado in Denver for acquiring the rotational acquisitions presented. We also gratefully acknowledge Robin de Paus, Philips Healthcare, for his preparation of the 2D StentBoost Subtract movies (Movies 1–4).

APPENDIX: SUPPLEMENTARY MATERIAL

Supplementary material can be found, in the online version, at doi:10.1016/j.ccl.2009.03.007.

REFERENCES

1. Cook S, Wenaweser P, Togni M, et al. Incomplete stent apposition and very late stent thrombosis after drug-eluting stent implantation. Circulation 2007; 115:2426–34.
2. Windecker S, Meier B. Late coronary stent thrombosis. Circulation 2007;116:1952–65.
3. Koolen JJ, van het Veer M, Hanekamp CEE. StentBoost image enhancement: first clinical experience. Medicamundi 2005;49(2):4–8.
4. Ross JC, Langan D, Manjeshwar R, et al. Registration and integration for fluoroscopy device enhancement. Med Image Comput Comput Assist Interv Int Conf Med Image Comput Comput Assist Interv 2005;8(Pt 1):851–8.
5. Perrenot B, Vaillant R, Prost R, et al. Motion compensation for 3D tomographic reconstruction of stent in x-ray cardiac rotational angiography. 3rd IEEE International Symposium on Biomedical Imaging, Arlington, VA. April 6–9, 2006:1224–7.
6. Perrenot B, Vaillant R, Prost R, et al. Motion correction for coronary stent reconstruction from rotational x-ray projection sequences. IEEE Trans Med Imaging 2007;26(10):1412–23.
7. Perrenot B, Vaillant R, Laurence G, et al. 3D motion compensated tomographic reconstruction of coronary stents from x-ray rotational sequence: an experimental study. EMBS 2007. 29th Annual International Conference of the IEEE, Lyon, France. August 22–26, 2007:735–8.

8. Ouled Zaid A, Hadded I, Belhaj W, et-al. Improved localization of coronary stents based on image enhancement. Int J Biomed Sci;4(3):212–6.

9. Schoonenberg G, Lelong P, Florent R, et al. The effect of automated marker detection on in vivo volumetric stent reconstruction. Med Image Comput Comput Assist Interv Int Conf Med Image Comput Comput Assist Interv 2008;11(Pt 2):87–94.

10. Bismuth V, Vaillant R. Elastic registration for stent enhancement in x-ray image sequences. ICIP; 2008. p. 2400–3.

11. Kompatsiaris I, Tzovaras D, Koutkias V, et al. Deformable boundary detection of stents in angiographic images. IEEE Trans Med Imaging 2000; 9(6):652–62.

12. Close RA, Abbey CK, Whiting JS. Improved localization of coronary stents using layer decomposition. Comput Aided Surg 2002;7:84–9.

13. Hanekamp CEE, Koolen JJ, Bonnier HJRM, et al. First clinical experience with Stent boost, a new image enhancement technique to improve stent visibility using regular x-ray exposure. In: van Ofwegen-Hanekamp CEE. Pathofysiology and clinical aspects of coronary stenting, Ph.D. thesis; ISBN: 90-9018830-4; 2004. p. 41–53.

14. Conway DSG, Smith WHT, Moore J, et al. Measurement of coronary stent expansion using StentBoost™ image enhancement software: a comparison with intravascular ultrasound. Br Heart J 2005;91(Supplement I):A39–40.

15. Mishell JM, Vakharia KT, Ports TA, et al. Determination of adequate coronary stent expansion using StentBoost™, a novel fluoroscopic image processing technique. Catheter Cardiovasc Interv 2007;69: 84–93.

16. Agostoni P, Verheye S, Vermeersch P, et al. "Virtual" in-vivo bench test for bifurcation stenting with "StentBoost". Int J Cardiol, 2009;133:e67–9.

17. Agostoni P, Verheye S. Bifurcation stenting with a dedicated biolimus-eluting stent: x-ray visual enhancement of the final angiographic result with "StentBoost Subtract™". Catheter Cardiovasc Interv 2007;70:233–6.

18. Garcia JA, Bakker NH, de Paus R, et al. StentBoost: a useful clinical tool. Medicamundi 2008;52(2).

19. Schoonenberg GAF, van den Houten PW, Florent R, et al. Device boosting using rotational x-ray angiography. SPIE 2009, to appear.

20. Gavit L, Carlier S, Hayase M, et al. The evolving role of coronary angiography and fluoroscopy in cardiac diagnosis and intervention. EuroInterv 2007;2: 526–32.

21. Movassaghi B, Schaefer D, Grass M, et al. 3D reconstruction of coronary stents in vivo based on motion compensated x-ray angiograms. In: Larsen R, Nielsen M, Sporring J, editors. MICCAI; 2006. LNCS 4191, p. 177–84.

22. Movassaghi B, Garcia JA, Schoonenberg G, et al. In vivo three-dimensional reconstruction of coronary stents based on motion compensated x-ray angiograms: first in human results. Am J Cardiol 2006; 98(8 Supplement 1):S104.

23. Schäfer D, Movassaghi B, Grass M, et al. Three-dimensional reconstruction of coronary stents in vivo based on motion compensated x-ray angiography. In: Medical imaging 2007: visualization and image-guided procedures. Cleary KR, Miga MI, editors. Proceedings of SPIE Vol. 6509 (SPIE, Bellingham, WA 2007) 65091M.

24. Betsou S, Efstathopoulos EP, Katritsis D, et al. Patient radiation doses during cardiac catheterization procedures. Br J Radiol 1998;71:634–9.

25. Fitzgerald PJ, Oshima A, Hayase M, et al. Final results of the Can Routine Ultrasound Influence Stent Expansion (CRUISE) study. Circulation 2000; 102(5):523–30.

Two and Three-Dimensional Quantitative Coronary Angiography

Ioannis Pantos, MSc[a,b], Efstathios P. Efstathopoulos, PhD[b],
Demosthenes G. Katritsis, MD, PhD, FRCP[a,*]

KEYWORDS

- Quantitative coronary analysis • Two dimensional
- Three dimensional

Contrast coronary angiography and left ventriculography are the most widely used methods for evaluating cardiac disease, especially coronary artery disease. Visual inspection of coronary angiograms has been traditionally used to appreciate the extent of coronary disease, and assessment of stenosis severity is the usual means by which coronary lesions are quantified.[1] Several experimental studies have shown that diameter percent stenosis, under carefully controlled conditions, provides a useful index of the significance of a coronary lesion.[2,3] However, the general applicability of this index, especially in the presence of diffuse disease affecting more than one vessel, has been seriously questioned.[1,4] Absolute measurements of arterial narrowing, such as mean and minimal coronary diameter, and of minimal cross-sectional area have also been used to assess stenosis severity, and have been shown to be better markers of progression or regression of coronary atherosclerosis.[5,6] In addition, subjective assessment of coronary lesions has been found to correlate poorly with pathoanatomic studies[7,8] and to suffer significant intraobserver and interobserver variability.[9–12] A precise method of lesion characterization and quantitation of arterial lumen dimensions from coronary angiograms is, therefore, necessary for the assessment of coronary disease and the efficacy of therapeutic procedures in the catheterization laboratory.

The last decades have witnessed significant progress in the development and evolution of quantitative methods, from the initial simplistic techniques to the present advanced three-dimensional (3D) systems. These systems are collectively known as quantitative coronary angiography (QCA) systems. Although methods for the assessment of the hemodynamic significance and composition of coronary atherosclerosis have evolved, the ability of QCA to provide objective dimensional assessment of coronary lesions is still useful and has led to its widespread application in both scientific research and clinical practice.

TWO-DIMENSIONAL QUANTITATIVE CORONARY ANGIOGRAPHY SYSTEMS

In the majority of systems used in clinical practice today, lesion quantitation is performed directly on angiographic images that are two-dimensional (2D) projections of the complex 3D structure of the arterial tree. The angiographer assesses the actual geometry of the arterial tree by acquiring images from different projection angles, and lesion quantification is performed on a single or multiple 2D views. Thus, these systems are termed *2D QCA systems* to distinguish them from the latest

This work is supported by a grant from the S. Niarchos Foundation.

[a] Department of Cardiology, Coronary Flow Research Unit, Athens Euroclinic, 9 Athanassiadou Street, 115 21 Athens, Greece

[b] Department of Radiology, Medical School, University of Athens, Rimini 1, Chaidari, 1246 Athens, Greece

* Corresponding author.

E-mail address: dkatritsis@euroclinic.gr (D.G. Katritsis).

Cardiol Clin 27 (2009) 491–502

doi:10.1016/j.ccl.2009.03.008

systems, which acquire the 3D geometry of the lesion and perform lesion quantitation on the reconstructed 3D lesion model. Earlier 2D QCA systems were based on computer-interactive visual interpretation of the coronary vessels, whereas newer ones are based on automated vessel extraction either by vessel-edge detection or densitometry techniques.

Quantitative Coronary Angiography by Computer-Interactive Visual Interpretation

Several studies have documented the large intraobserver and interobserver variability that results from subjective visual grading of coronary stenotic lesions.[9–12] Moreover, by this technique, the degree of luminal narrowing can be determined only in terms of percentage diameter stenosis assessed from one or more views. Initial efforts to quantify arterial dimensions and increase accuracy and reproducibility of visual assessment of coronary artery disease resulted in the introduction of systems involving computer-interactive visual interpretation. These early QCA systems were based on digital calipers or computer-assisted lesion reconstruction.

Digital calipers
The earliest computer-interactive QCA systems employed a projector that displayed cursors on the screen to define certain image points.[13] Two-point distances across the projected angiographic lumen defined minimum and normal vessel diameter, which were electronically computed, as was percent stenosis. A modification of the above approach used handheld calipers wired to a programmable calculator to measure and record local vessel diameter from the projector screen and to compute percent stenosis.[14] Digital calipers did not overcome the limitations of visual estimates of percent diameter stenosis. Subsequent studies revealed that they systematically underestimated severe stenoses (>75%) and overestimated less severe stenoses (<75%), while the reproducibility of the method was poor.[15]

Computer-assisted image reconstruction
Following digital caliper analyses, the next advance in QCA systems was introduced by the cardiovascular computation laboratory at the University of Washington.[16] This system attempted to compensate for three potential sources of error in the analysis of cinefilms: (1) the difference in lesion dimensions among angiographic projections, (2) pincushion distortion causing increased magnification of objects viewed in the periphery of the angiographic field, and (3) divergence of the x-ray beam with consequent distortion of the

image due to selective magnification of objects that are closest to the x-ray source.[17] Two perpendicular views of the diseased segment were projected at high (×5) magnification, and the borders of the angiographic lumen were manually traced from the "normal" proximal portion, through the stenosis, to the "normal" distal portion. The borders were digitized and the lesion image was converted to true scale by a computer program corrected for x-ray beam divergence and pincushion distortion using the catheter as a scaling device. The orthogonal images were matched at the minimal diameter and combined to form a 3D representation that assumes elliptical lesion geometry. From the composite image, absolute dimensions, percent diameter stenosis, and atheroma mass were calculated. The major weakness of the method, as with digital calipers, is that it is based on the image-processing capabilities of the human eye and brain to locate the border of the lumen image. In addition, the method is slow and labor-intensive, often taking more than 10 minutes for the analysis of a given stenosis.[18]

Quantitative Coronary Angiography with Automated Lumen Border Definition

The majority of QCA systems currently used in clinical practice feature automated lumen border definition. Most of the available systems nowadays are based on vessel edge detection algorithms to designate the arterial lumen on the coronary angiogram. Earlier systems combined edge detection with densitometric techniques or used densitometry alone.

Densitometry
Densitometry is based on the Beer-Lambert law, which states that the logarithmic attenuation of an x-ray beam through a vessel is proportional to the thickness of the contrast inside that vessel.[19] When a straight vessel is viewed perpendicular to its central axis, the integration of the background-subtracted attenuation profile provides a value directly proportional to lumen cross-sectional area. A direct estimate of percent area reduction can be found by comparing this area estimate in a stenosis with that at a nearby normal vessel segment. With proper image scaling it is also possible to estimate absolute area reduction. Densitometry is performed by manually defining regions of interest (ROIs) on the angiographic image. One ROI is placed across the stenotic segment, another ROI is placed across the normal segment, and two ROIs are placed on both sides outside the arterial lumen to acquire the average background density.

Theoretically, densitometry avoids many of the problems associated with stenoses having a non-cylindrical geometry. Densitometric analysis is particularly suited for the analysis of eccentric lesions because the measured signal reflects the amount of contrast medium within the stenosis independently of its geometry, and the measured degree of stenosis is the same for any angiographic projection perpendicular to the long axis of the lesion.[20] Therefore, analysis in a single projection is sufficient for calculating the degree of stenosis. Accurate assessment of asymmetric lesion is theoretically useful in the case of percutaneous coronary intervention because the mechanical disruption of the internal artery wall, caused by the procedure, leads to eccentric, asymmetric morphologic changes.[21,22] An additional advantage of densitometry is that it is independent of image resolution (blur or unsharpness), unlike edge-detection methods, which tend to overestimate vessel diameter in the presence of motion unsharpness.[23]

Application of densitometry in clinical practice has exposed the problems of the technique due to various error sources. Densitometry is much more sensitive than edge detection to densitometric nonlinearities that occur due to the polyenergetic x-ray beam, image-intensifier characteristics, and such phenomena as vignetting and veil glare.[24,25] Errors also occur when the lesion is not perpendicular to the x-ray beam (foreshortening vessel) and when the lesion overlaps with other structures. Finally, the method is based on several premises that are not always valid in clinical practice: It is assumed, but not always true, that radiographic magnification is uniform, radiographic exposure for a single frame is also uniform, and, most importantly, contrast distribution is equal in both the normal and stenotic arterial segments.[21] The method has inherent limitations. Few investigators have demonstrated close agreement of densitometric results from different views taken from the some vessel.[26] Others investigators have reported important discrepancies between densitometric evaluation in different views.[11,27,28]

The reliability of densitometric assessments of luminal dimensions is now considered inferior to that of geometric coronary measurements.[29] Consequently, densitometry did not follow the substantial evolution of more accurate edge-detection algorithms embedded into new generations of QCA systems.[30,31]

Vessel-edge detection

First-generation systems Vessel images have edge gradients rather than sharply demarcated edges.

Thus, various computerized methods using specific edge-detection algorithms to locate spatially disparate points within the edge gradient have been developed. The first attempts at computerized analysis of digitized radiographic images were made at the Biomedical Image Analysis Laboratory of the Jet Propulsion Laboratory in conjunction with the University of Southern California School of Medicine.[32] Initial methods for automated operator-interactive definition of lumen borders were developed by Sanders and colleagues[33] and Alderman and colleagues[34] in the late 70s and early 80s. Subsequent QCA systems that incorporated automated edge detection were introduced in the mid- and late 80s by the Erasmus University (CAAS [Cardiovascular Angiography Analysis System]),[35] the University of Michigan (Artrek),[36] Duke University (DUQUES [Duke University Quantitative/Qualitative Catheterization Evaluation System,[37]]) and the Stuttgart Biomedical Institute.[38] The later system is actually a member of a series of QCA systems that combined densitometry with edge detection. Other systems that combined the two methods were developed by Collins and colleagues,[39] Kirkeeide and colleagues,[40] and Pfaff and colleagues.[41] This approach was extensively investigated on both diagnostic and intervention coronary angiograms at St. Thomas' Hospital, London, in the mid-80s.[11,12,27,28] **Fig. 1** illustrates a representative coronary analysis by a system that incorporates both edge detection and densitometry.

A coronary analysis procedure with all these QCA systems entails film digitization (in the case of cineangiograms), image calibration, and contour detection. For digitization, the cinefilm is mounted on a cine-video converter and projected onto a high-resolution video camera, which digitizes the selected cineframes. Calibration is performed by using the catheter as a scaling device. The edge-detection procedure is initiated by manually defining the proximal and distal segments of the vessel that contains the stenosis. The vessel centerline is automatically defined. Then, linear density profiles (scanlines) are generated perpendicular to the centerline over the entire segment length. The first and second derivatives of these density profiles are computed and the contours along the segment are defined by the application of the so-called "minimal cost criterion" to a weighted sum of the first and second derivative functions.[18] The quantitative data obtained by these QCA systems are minimal obstruction diameter, extend of obstruction, percent diameter stenosis, percent area stenosis, mean

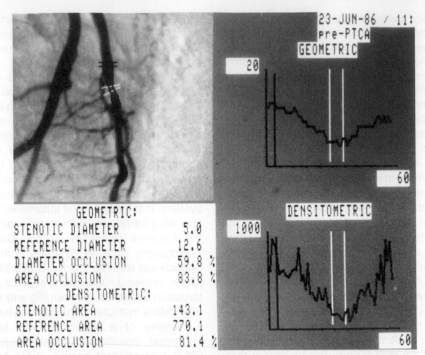

GEOMETRIC:
STENOTIC DIAMETER   5.0
REFERENCE DIAMETER   12.6
DIAMETER OCCLUSION   59.8 %
AREA OCCLUSION   83.8 %
DENSITOMETRIC:
STENOTIC AREA   143.1
REFERENCE AREA   770.1
AREA OCCLUSION   81.4 %

23-JUN-86 / 11:
pre-PTCA
GEOMETRIC
20
60
DENSITOMETRIC
1000
60

Fig. 1. Representative coronary analysis displaying quantitative data performed with a QCA system combining geometric (edge detection) and densitometric methods. (*Courtesy of* D.G. Katritsis, MD, Athens, Greece. Assessment of the results of coronary angioplasty by computer-assisted quantitation on digital subtraction angiograms. Presented at the University of London Department of Cardiology. London, 1990; with permission.)

diameter of nonobstructed coronary segments, plaque mass, and lesion symmetry.

Second-generation systems All systems previously mentioned are considered first-generation systems and have been shown to provide fairly reliable assessment of coronary dimensions.[42] However, several investigators have demonstrated that a major error frequently observed with these systems was the overestimation of sizes of small (<1 mm diameter) vessels.[43] The vessel size below which overestimation occurs and the degree of overestimation are related to the focal spot size of the imaging chain. The phenomenon can be explained in terms of the point-spread function of the respective imaging chain.[31] This posed an important limitation for meaningful QCA analysis because evidence had showed that analysis of absolute coronary dimensions is more appropriate for the assessment of therapeutic interventions and that the minimal luminal diameter is the greatest single determinant of the hemodynamic impact of coronary narrowing.[23,44] Therefore, a new generation of QCA systems has emerged incorporating correction algorithms to overcome these systematic limitations. These second-generation systems corrected vessel overestimation and significantly improved accuracy in the submillimeter range

over the entire range of coronary dimension. Small coronary diameters (as little as 0.5 mm) could be analyzed more accurately with these systems.[31] It has been shown that it is reasonable to aim for precision values of 0.10 mm to 0.14 mm or less for in vitro analyses and 0.20 mm or less for in vivo analyses.[45] The observed precision values in second-generation systems for arteries 1 mm in diameter or narrower were worse than the overall precision values, thus the gain of accuracy in these system is accompanied by loss of precision in the submillimeter range.[31] **Fig. 2** illustrates a representative lesion analysis with a second-generation system (QCA-CMS, Medis, The Netherlands).

Third-generation systems A subsequent development in cardiovascular x-ray imaging systems with an impact on QCA systems was the introduction of digital flat-panel detectors instead of the conventional image intensifier–based systems. Flat-panel–based images do not significantly influence QCA results and thus no further optimization of the edge-detection algorithm is necessary.[46] However, to exploit the redundancy of information of flat-panel detector images, a new, third generation of QCA systems was developed. These systems employ gradient field transform detection algorithms.[47,48] With gradient field transform, the changes in brightness between points in an image

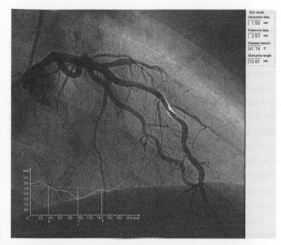

Fig. 2. Representative analysis of a left anterior descending coronary lesion displaying quantitative data by a second-generation QCA system. (*Courtesy of* Athens Euroclinic, Coronary Flow Research Unit, QCA-CMS, Medis, The Netherlands.)

are assessed from all directions. By contrast, minimal-cost algorithms assess brightness only perpendicularly to the centerline of the vessel.[30] Third-generation systems are more adequate for assessing smaller diameters[47] and more capable of tracing irregular borders. Such systems are therefore particularly suitable for the quantification of complex coronary lesions.[48] Overestimation of small diameters is thought to be due to low contrast concentration in small vessels and to the point spread function of the x-ray imaging chain. Thus, third-generation systems, in addition to offering the benefits of fully digital image acquisition and superior image quality of flat-panel detector images, also make for more accurate estimations of small diameters compared with second-generation systems, although the problem of overestimation is not completely eliminated.[47]

THREE-DIMENSIONAL QUANTITATIVE CORONARY ANGIOGRAPHY SYSTEMS

Significant advances have made QCA systems more accurate and precise. However, all QCA systems mentioned so far require operators to rely on 2D silhouettes to interpret the 3D structure of the vessel. The combination of vessel overlap, suboptimal projections, and individual anatomic variation may result in insufficient 2D images and may partially account for the suboptimal sensitivity and specificity of coronary angiography or lead to inaccurate QCA analysis.[49] Indeed, foreshortening of vessel segments ranges from 0% to 50% depending on the coronary artery and the vessel segment within the artery even for "optimal" views

selected by experienced interventional cardiologists.[50,51] Additionally, 2D images can provide only quantitative evaluation of such features as bifurcation angles between main and side branches and vessel curvature.[52] Thus, in bifurcation lesions, 2D QCA cannot provide baseline anatomic differences (eg, vessel size, bifurcation angle) useful in helping the interventional cardiologist determine the best bifurcation intervention technique.[53,54] To overcome the disadvantages of 2D quantitative measures, 3D QCA systems were introduced. They use the detected vessel contours in two projections to visualize a 3D model of the arterial segment and perform quantitative analysis on the generated 3D modeling image.

Three-Dimensional Coronary Artery Modeling

The process of 3D QCA analysis does not differ significantly from 2D analysis. Three-dimensional analysis requires acquisition of two angiographic views that (1) differ by an angle of at least 30° and that (2) display the lesion with no or minimal overlap. Image calibration is performed either by using the catheter as a scaling device or is automatically based on the DICOM (Digital Imaging and Communications in Medicine standard for distributing and viewing medical images) information in the images. Once calibrated, the two views are used to create the 3D vessel image. Depending on the system, this is achieved by either marking a point proximally, distally, and at the stenosis on both views, or by defining a common image point (a landmark common to both images) and two points distal and proximal to the stenotic region.[55,56] The software automatically creates the contours of the vessels in the two views and in the 3D model of the coronary artery. Operators can focus on, zoom in on, and rotate the generated 3D vessel segment.[55] The software determines minimum luminal diameter and area, proximal and distal reference diameters and areas, percentage of diameter and area stenosis, and lesion length. The 3D model of arterial segment is available in real time and the technique does not require alteration of the sequence of catheterization, extra angiographic views, or contrast injections.[55] Once two appropriate views are obtained in standard angiography, the 3D model is obtainable. This enables the angiographer to appreciate the complex arterial curvilinear structure and to select the optimal angiographic view with the least vessel overlap and least foreshortening in the region of interest.[52] This view can be used for potential coronary intervention while stent size and length can be chosen by the quantitative data of the analyzed lesion. Three-dimensional modeling and analysis of bifurcations are also possible. In this case, both the main branch and the side branch are analyzed and the bifurcation angle is also provided. **Figs. 3** and **4** illustrate representative models of arterial segments and subsequent quantitative analysis with two 3D QCA systems.

Commercially Available Three-dimensional Quantitative Coronary Angiography Systems

Three-dimensional QCA systems became commercially available very recently and clinical experience is limited.

The first 3D QCA system that became commercially available (CardiOp-B, Paieon Medical Ltd., Park Afek, Israel) was validated against a 2D QCA system (Medview, Medcom Telemedicine Technology, Tel Aviv, Israel). Three-dimensional modeling and analysis appears to be feasible in all attempted angiograms requiring between 4 and 30 minutes to perform, and the precision of 3D QCA is superior to that of 2D QCA in the measurement of minimal lesion diameter, minimal lesion area, and lesion length.[52] In another study, CardiOp-B was evaluated by correlating the measured proximal and distal stent diameters and stent length with the predefined size of the stents at the used inflation pressure. Although high linear correlation to predefined stent sizes was reported for all measures, the true proximal and distal stent diameters were slightly underestimated while length of the stent was accurately

measured.[55] In vivo evaluation of CardiOp-B against a second-generation 2D QCA system (CAAS II)[29,30] has confirmed the good correlation between luminal diameter measurements and phantom actual diameter values for both systems.[57] However, both systems significantly underestimated the actual phantom diameters and CardiOp-B demonstrated poorer accuracy in diameter measurement compared with the 2D system, contradicting the results of a previous study.[52] The investigators attributed the discrepancy to the use of a validated and presumably more accurate 2D QCA system to evaluate in their comparison with CardiOp-B.[57]

Following the introduction of the first 3D QCA system, another system became available. This is 3D-CA (Philips Medical Systems Nederland BV, Best, The Netherlands), which was tested on images acquired by rotational coronary angiography.[58,59] In the case of rotational angiography, the orthogonal, electrocardiography-gated views are acquired through a cine run during which the gantry is rotated by 110°, paying attention to maintain optimal opacification of the coronary vessels for the time required (4 seconds) by the gantry to complete its rotation.[60] Quantitative analysis of this 3D QCA system was evaluated against a second-generation 2D QCA system (CAAS II),[29,30] while an intracoronary guide wire with radiopaque markers provided the "gold standard" for length measurements. Three-dimensional QCA provided more accurate information on coronary arterial segment length than 2D QCA, without

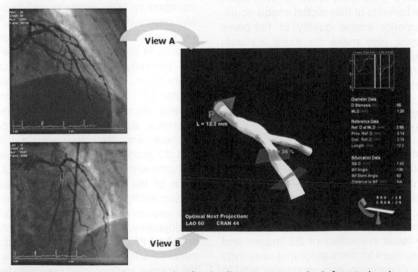

Fig. 3. Representative 3D modeling and analysis by the CardiOp-B system of a left anterior descending–diagonal bifurcation lesion. At the left side of the figure are the two "orthogonal" angiographic views used to create the 3D model of the bifurcation. (*From* Schlundt C, Kreft JG, Fuchs F, et al. Three-dimensional on-line reconstruction of coronary bifurcated lesions to optimize side-branch stenting. Catheter Cardiovasc Interv 2006;68(2):249–53; with permission.)

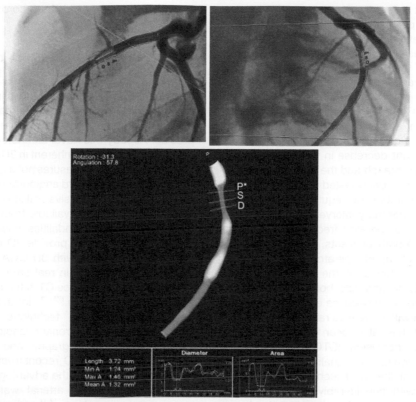

Fig. 4. Representative 3D modeling and analysis by the CAAS 5 system applied to a stenotic phantom wedged in a porcine left coronary artery. The upper side of the picture shows the two "orthogonal" angiographic views used to generate the 3D model of the artery. (*From* Ramcharitar S, Daeman J, Patterson M, et al. First direct in vivo comparison of two commercially available three-dimensional quantitative coronary angiography systems. Catheter Cardiovasc Interv 2008;71(1):44–50; with permission.)

differences in reference vessel diameter estimation. Interestingly, the angiographic view selected according to the operator's expertise as the best representative of the segment of interest often differed significantly from the least foreshortening view automatically generated by the 3D QCA system.[60]

Recently, CardiOp-B was compared in vivo with a newly introduced 3D QCA system (CAAS 5, Pie Medical Imaging, Maastricht, The Netherlands) by using phantoms of known luminal diameters. Qualitative assessment of the minimum, maximum, and mean luminal diameters and the minimal luminal areas showed that CardiOp-B significantly underestimated the minimum luminal diameter while both systems significantly overestimated the maximum luminal diameter and the minimal lumen area over the phantom's true value.[61] The degree of accuracy and precision in both the luminal and area measurements was greater for CAAS 5.[61] Discrepancy of results between the two systems was attributed to differences in image calibration and efficiency of the edge-detection algorithm:

CardiOp-B uses manual image calibration with the catheter as a scaling device while CAAS 5 automatically calibrates the image using the DICOM information. Manual calibration poses a potential limitation because it has been reported that if the catheter is not in the same plane as the evaluated vessel segment, this method can give rise to differences in magnification and influence the accuracy of analysis.[62] With CardiOp-B, the detected contour deviated significantly from the vessel's edge. As a result, automatically generated contours often had to be manually corrected. Thus, it was noted, automatic edge detection was not equally accurate for both systems.[61]

Clinical Applications

In clinical practice, 3D QCA can reliably assess absolute coronary luminal diameter and length as well as bifurcation anatomy and aid the operator with therapeutic interventions, such as stent implantation. Another potential advantage of 3D QCA that has to be clinically validated is the improvement of procedural success rates in chronic total occlusions.

Two studies have used CardiOp-B to evaluate bifurcation lesions.[53,54] These studies confirmed the ability of the system to create the main and bifurcation branch and acquire the relative dimensions of the proximal main branch, distal main branch, side branch, and branch angulation. Moreover, an anatomic change that occurs in a bifurcation was reported: After stenting, there was a significant decrease in the angle between the distal main branch and the side branch.[53]

CardiOp-B has been tested for choice of stent length and number of required stents during percutaneous coronary intervention. It was found that experienced operators frequently misinterpret the required length of stents, and that 3D QCA would have changed operator decision-making regarding the choice of the appropriate stent length.[51] This finding has both procedural and economic relevance because excess stent length is associated with increased rates of restenosis.[63]

CardiOp-B has also been used to evaluate chronic total occlusion (CTO) lesions of the coronary arteries. Recanalization of CTOs remains one of the most technically challenging procedures with considerably lower procedural success rates than other lesion subsets.[64,65] Off-line analysis with a 2D QCA system (Medcon Telemedicine Technology, McKesson, San Francisco, California) and CardiOp-B revealed that 3D QCA yielded significantly smaller area of stenosis and shorter lesion length, the later presumably due to inaccurate 2D measurements.[66] Three-dimensional modeling of CTOs can clearly image the stump area, delineate the lesion path, and, in certain occasions of late arterial filling, provide information for precise calculation of the severity of the stenosis and lesion length. Thus, 3D modeling may serve as a useful tool for planning interventional procedures for CTOs and improve their success rates.[66]

A novel clinical application of CardiOp-B is its integration into a recently developed magnetic navigation system in which physicians operate a computer interface that controls the magnetic field produced by two magnets positioned on either side of the fluoroscopic table.[67,68] The magnetic field creates a magnetic vector that determines the orientation of the guide-wire tip as it is advanced through the coronary anatomy. The 3D virtual vessel roadmap is created by the 3D reconstruction software (CardiOp-B) and the system computes the navigation plan from the reconstructed virtual path that supplies all the vectors required to navigate the guide wire through the artery, even if the coronary anatomy is complex or extremely tortuous.

Three-dimensional Quantitative Coronary Angiography Systems in Perspective

Only very recently introduced into clinical practice, 3D QCA systems have the potential, with further development, to become even more accurate and precise. Already this novel technology has solved many of the limitations inherent in 2D QCA systems and provides lesion measures not available with 2D imaging. Unlike standard angiographic images, 3D modeling is comprehensive as it integrates into one image all information available from angiography. Some other imaging modalities, such as multislice CT and MRI, can also provide 3D arterial reconstructions. However, with 3D QCA systems, the 3D image is available in real time. An additional advantage over multislice CT is the reduced mean effective patient dose.[69–71] Intravascular ultrasound is an imaging technique that can be performed during coronary angiography. The combination of angiography and intravascular ultrasound provides 3D reconstructions of coronary arteries that offer the advantage of including reconstruction of the arterial wall.[72] However, acquisition and analysis of the intravascular ultrasound data set represents an invasive approach that takes additional time and costs, while the fusion image is available only off line.

Finally, 3D QCA, by generating a 3D coronary model, can provide important anatomic characteristics of the arterial tree, such as vessel curvature, vessel torsion, and bifurcation take-off angles, that may not be reliably assessed through 2D angiographic images.[73,74] All these anatomic features have been correlated with hemodynamic parameters that may potentially affect development of atherosclerosis and probably plaque rupture.[75,76] Hemodynamic studies of the coronary arteries are particularly challenging because of the small size of the coronary vessels, their tortuous course, and their attachment to contracting myocardium. Important hemodynamic quantities, such as wall shear stress, cannot be accurately accessed in vivo in the coronary tree by current imaging modalities, such as phase-contrast MRI, ultrasound, and pulsed Doppler ultrasound, because of their limited spatial and temporal resolution.[77] Alternatively, computational fluid dynamics have been used by various investigators to study the hemodynamic parameters potentially involved in coronary artery disease.[78–80] In the case of computational fluid dynamics studies, 3D coronary reconstruction can provide patient-specific coronary geometries for which pressure and

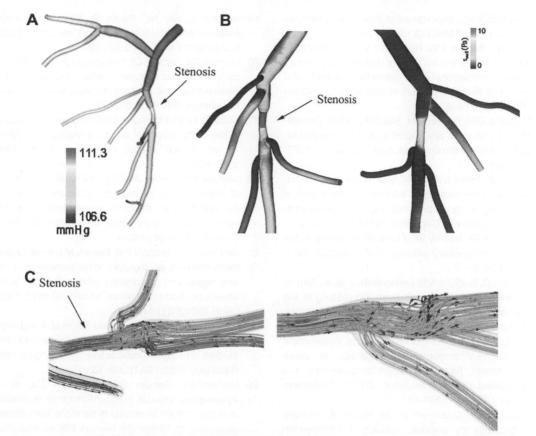

Fig. 5. Computational fluid dynamic study of stenotic flow on a patient-specific coronary geometry generated in 3D. (*A*) Pressure distribution in mm Hg. (*B*) Wall shear stress distribution in pascals (Pa) as seen from two different views. (*C*) Streamlines in the location downstream of the stenosis as seen from two different views (*Courtesy of Athens Euroclinic, Coronary Flow Research Unit.*)

velocity components of flow are calculated by the numerical solution of the governing equations of fluid flow (**Fig. 5**).

SUMMARY

QCA has undergone substantial evolution from simplistic computer-assisted methods of visual interpretation of coronary angiograms to recently introduced systems incorporating 3D modeling and quantitative analysis algorithms. The ability of QCA to provide objective dimensional assessment of coronary lesions is still useful and has led to its widespread application in both scientific research and clinical practice. Most of the currently available systems are based on vessel edge detection algorithms to designate the arterial lumen on conventional, 2D coronary angiograms. The recent development of 3D QCA may solve many of the limitations inherent in 2D QCA and provides coronary artery assessment capabilities not available with 2D imaging.

REFERENCES

1. Marcus ML, Harrison DG, White CW, et al. Assessing the physiologic significance of coronary obstructions in patients: importance of diffuse undetected atherosclerosis. Prog Cardiovasc Dis 1988;31(1): 39–56.
2. Gould KL, Lipscomb K, Hamilton GW. Physiologic basis for assessing critical coronary stenosis. Instantaneous flow response and regional distribution during coronary hyperemia as measures of coronary flow reserve. Am J Cardiol 1974;33(1): 87–94.
3. Lipscomb K, Gould KL. Mechanism of the effect of coronary artery stenosis on coronary flow in the dog. Am Heart J 1975;89(1):60–7.
4. Marcus ML, Skorton DJ, Johnson MR, et al. Visual estimates of percent diameter coronary stenosis: "a battered gold standard". J Am Coll Cardiol 1988;11(4):882–5.
5. White CW, Wright CB, Doty DB, et al. Does visual interpretation of the coronary arteriogram predict

the physiologic importance of a coronary stenosis? N Engl J Med 1984;310(13):819–24.

6. Wijns W, Serruys PW, Reiber JH, et al. Quantitative angiography of the left anterior descending coronary artery: correlations with pressure gradient and results of exercise thallium scintigraphy. Circulation 1985;71(2):273–9.

7. Hutchins GM, Bulkley BH, Ridolfi RL, et al. Correlation of coronary arteriograms and left ventriculograms with postmortem studies. Circulation 1977; 56(1):32–7.

8. Isner JM, Kishel J, Kent KM, et al. Accuracy of angiographic determination of left main coronary arterial narrowing. Angiographic–histologic correlative analysis in 28 patients. Circulation 1981;63(5):1056–64.

9. DeRouen TA, Murray JA, Owen W. Variability in the analysis of coronary arteriograms. Circulation 1977; 55(2):324–8.

10. Fisher LD, Judkins MP, Lesperance J, et al. Reproducibility of coronary arteriographic reading in the Coronary Artery Surgery Study (CASS). Cathet Cardiovasc Diagn 1982;8(6):565–75.

11. Katritsis D, Lythall DA, Cooper IC, et al. Assessment of coronary angioplasty: comparison of visual assessment, hand-held caliper measurement and automated digital quantitation. Cathet Cardiovasc Diagn 1988;15(4):237–42.

12. Katritsis D. Assessment of the results of coronary angioplasty by computer-assisted quantitation on digital subtraction angiograms. London: Department of Cardiology, St Thomas' Hospital, University of London; 1990.

13. Gensini GG, Kelly AE, Da Costa BC, et al. Quantitative angiography: the measurement of coronary vasomobility in the intact animal and man. Chest 1971; 60(6):522–30.

14. Scoblionko DP, Brown BG, Mitten S, et al. A new digital electronic caliper for measurement of coronary arterial stenosis: comparison with visual estimates and computer-assisted measurements. Am J Cardiol 1984;53(6):689–93.

15. Kalbfleisch SJ, McGillem MJ, Pinto IM, et al. Comparison of automated quantitative coronary angiography with caliper measurements of percent diameter stenosis. Am J Cardiol 1990;65(18):1181–4.

16. Brown BG, Bolson E, Frimer M, et al. Quantitative coronary arteriography: estimation of dimensions, hemodynamic resistance, and atheroma mass of coronary artery lesions using the arteriogram and digital computation. Circulation 1977;55(2):329–37.

17. Katritsis D, Webb-Peploe M. Limitations of coronary angiography: an underestimated problem? Clin Cardiol 1991;14(1):20–4.

18. Hermiller JB, Cusma JT, Spero LA, et al. Quantitative and qualitative coronary angiographic analysis: review of methods, utility, and limitations. Cathet Cardiovasc Diagn 1992;25(2):110–31.

19. Sandor T, Als AV, Paulin S. Cine-densitometric measurement of coronary arterial stenoses. Cathet Cardiovasc Diagn 1979;5(3):229–45.

20. Nichols AB, Gabrieli CF, Fenoglio JJ Jr, et al. Quantification of relative coronary arterial stenosis by cinevideodensitometric analysis of coronary arteriograms. Circulation 1984;69(3):512–22.

21. Katritsis D, Webb-Peploe MM. Angiographic quantitation of the results of coronary angioplasty: Where do we stand? Cathet Cardiovasc Diagn 1990; 21(2):65–71.

22. Serruys PW, Reiber JH, Wijns W, et al. Assessment of percutaneous transluminal coronary angioplasty by quantitative coronary angiography: diameter versus densitometric area measurements. Am J Cardiol 1984;54(6):482–8.

23. de Feyter PJ, Serruys PW, Davies MJ, et al. Quantitative coronary angiography to measure progression and regression of coronary atherosclerosis. Value, limitations, and implications for clinical trials. Circulation 1991;84(1):412–23.

24. Shaw CG, Ergun DL, Myerowitz PD, et al. A technique of scatter and glare correction for videodensitometric studies in digital subtraction videoangiography. Radiology 1982;142(1):209–13.

25. Reiber JH, Serruys PW, Kooijman CJ, et al. Approaches towards standardization in acquisition and quantitation of arterial dimensions from cineangiograms. In: Reiber JH, Serruys PW, editors. State of the art in quantitative coronary arteriography. Dordrecht: Martinus Nijhofff Publishers; 1986. p. 154–72.

26. Sanz ML, Mancini J, LeFree MT, et al. Variability of quantitative digital subtraction coronary angiography before and after percutaneous transluminal coronary angioplasty. Am J Cardiol 1987;60(1): 55–60.

27. Katritsis D, Lythall DA, Anderson MH, et al. Assessment of coronary angioplasty by an automated digital angiographic method. Am Heart J 1988; 116(5 Pt 1):1181–7.

28. Katritsis D, Webb-Peploe MM. Cardiac phase-related variability of border detection or densitometric quantitation of postangioplasty lumens. Am Heart J 1990;120(3):537–43.

29. Haase J, Escaned J, van Swijndregt EM, et al. Experimental validation of geometric and densitometric coronary measurements on the new generation Cardiovascular Angiography Analysis System (CAAS II). Cathet Cardiovasc Diagn 1993;30(2): 104–14.

30. Gronenschild E, Janssen J, Tijdens F. CAAS. II: a second generation system for off-line and on-line quantitative coronary angiography. Cathet Cardiovasc Diagn 1994;33(1):61–75.

31. Hausleiter J, Jost S, Nolte CW, et al. Comparative in-vitro validation of eight first- and second-generation

quantitative coronary angiography systems. Coron Artery Dis 1997;8(2):83–90.

32. Slezer RH, Blankenhorn DH, Crawford DW, et al. Computer analysis of cardiovascular imaginery. Paper presented at: Caltech/JPL Conference on Image Processing Technology, Data Sources and Software for Commercial and Scientific Applications; 3-5 Nov., 1976; Pasadena.

33. Sanders WJ, Alderman EL, Harrison DG. Coronary artery quantitation using digital image processing techniques. Comput Cardiol 1979;7: 15–20.

34. Alderman EL, Berte LE, Harrison DC, et al. Quantitation of coronary artery dimensions using digital image processing. In: Proceedings of SPIE. Stanford University: Stanford, USA; 1981. p. 273–8.

35. Reiber JH, Serruys PW, Kooijman CJ, et al. Assessment of short-, medium-, and long-term variations in arterial dimensions from computer-assisted quantitation of coronary cineangiograms. Circulation 1985;71(2):280–8.

36. Mancini GB, Simon SB, McGillem MJ, et al. Automated quantitative coronary arteriography: morphologic and physiologic validation in vivo of a rapid digital angiographic method. Circulation 1987;5(2):452–60.

37. Cusma JT, Spero LA, Hanemann JD, et al. A multiuser environment for the display and processing of digital cardiac angiographic images. In: Proceedings of SPIE. Newport Beach, USA; 1990. p. 310–20.

38. Barth JD, Faust U, Epple E. The objective measurement of coronary obstructions by digital image processing. Paper presented at: IEEE Conference on Physics and Engineering in Medical Imaging. Asilomar, USA, June 10–12, 1982.

39. Collins SM, Skorton DJ, Harrison DG, et al. Quantitative computer-based video densitometry and the physiological significance of coronary stenosis. Comput Cardiol 1982;10:219–22.

40. Kirkeeide R, Smalling RW, Gould KL. Automated measurement of artery diameter from arteriograms [Abstract]. Circulation 1982;55(Suppl II):325.

41. Pfaff JM, Whiting J, Vas R, et al. Automated geometric/densitometric coronary analysis: Comparison of accuracy and reproducibility [Abstract]. J Am Coll Cardiol 1985;5:501.

42. Spears JR, Sandor T, Als AV, et al. Computerized image analysis for quantitative measurement of vessel diameter from cineangiograms. Circulation 1983;68(2):453–61.

43. Herrington DM, Siebes M, Walford GD. Sources of error in quantitative coronary angiography. Cathet Cardiovasc Diagn 1993;29(4):314–21.

44. Gould KL. Dynamic coronary stenosis. Am J Cardiol 1980;45(2):286–92.

45. Reiber JH, Koning G, von Land CD, et al. Why and how should QCA systems by validated? In: Reiber JH, Serruys PW, editors. Progress in quantitative coronary arteriography. Dordrecht: Kluwer Academic Publishers; 1994. p. 33–48.

46. Tuinenburg JC, Koning G, Seppenwoolde Y, et al. Is there an effect of flat-panel-based imaging systems on quantitative coronary and vascular angiography? Catheter Cardiovasc Interv 2006;68(4):561–6.

47. Van Herck PL, Gavit L, Gorissen P, et al. Quantitative coronary arteriography on digital flat-panel system. Catheter Cardiovasc Interv 2004;63(2):192–200.

48. van der Zwet PM, Reiber JH. A new approach for the quantification of complex lesion morphology: the gradient field transform; basic principles and validation results. J Am Coll Cardiol 1994;24(1):216–24.

49. Thomas AC, Davies MJ, Dilly S, et al. Potential errors in the estimation of coronary arterial stenosis from clinical arteriography with reference to the shape of the coronary arterial lumen. Br Heart J 1986; 55(2):129–39.

50. Green NE, Chen SY, Hansgen AR, et al. Angiographic views used for percutaneous coronary interventions: a three-dimensional analysis of physician-determined vs. computer-generated views. Catheter Cardiovasc Interv 2005,64(4):451–9.

51. Gollapudi RR, Valencia R, Lee SS, et al. Utility of three-dimensional reconstruction of coronary angiography to guide percutaneous coronary intervention. Catheter Cardiovasc Interv 2007;69(4): 479–82.

52. Dvir D, Marom H, Guetta V, et al. Three-dimensional coronary reconstruction from routine single-plane coronary angiograms: in vivo quantitative validation. Int J Cardiovasc Intervent 2005;7(3):141–5.

53. Dvir D, Marom H, Assali A, et al. Bifurcation lesions in the coronary arteries: early experience with a novel 3-dimensional imaging and quantitative analysis before and after stenting. EuroInterv 2007;3:95–9.

54. Schlundt C, Kreft JG, Fuchs F, et al. Three-dimensional on-line reconstruction of coronary bifurcated lesions to optimize side-branch stenting. Catheter Cardiovasc Interv 2006;68(2):249–53.

55. Gradaus R, Mathies K, Breithardt G, et al. Clinical assessment of a new real time 3D quantitative coronary angiography system: evaluation in stented vessel segments. Catheter Cardiovasc Interv 2006; 68(1):44–9.

56. Green NE, Chen SY, Messenger JC, et al. Three-dimensional vascular angiography. Curr Probl Cardiol 2004;29(3):104–42.

57. Tsuchida K, van der Giessen W, Patterson M, et al. In vivo validation of a novel three-dimensional quantitative coronary angiography system (CardiOp-B™): comparison with a conventional two-dimensional system (CAAS II™) and with special reference to optical coherence tomography. EuroInterv 2007;3: 100–8.

58. Garcia JA, Chen J, Hansgen A, et al. Rotational angiography (RA) and three-dimensional imaging

(3-DRA): an available clinical tool. Int J Cardiovasc Imaging 2007;23(1):9–13.

59. Raman SV, Morford R, Neff M, et al. Rotational x-ray coronary angiography. Catheter Cardiovasc Interv 2004;63(2):201–7.

60. Agostoni P, Biondi-Zoccai G, Van Langenhove G, et al. Comparison of assessment of native coronary arteries by standard versus three-dimensional coronary angiography. Am J Cardiol 2008;102(3):272–9.

61. Ramcharitar S, Daeman J, Patterson M, et al. First direct in vivo comparison of two commercially available three-dimensional quantitative coronary angiography systems. Catheter Cardiovasc Interv 2008;71(1):44–50.

62. Fortin DF, Spero LA, Cusma JT, et al. Pitfalls in the determination of absolute dimensions using angiographic catheters as calibration devices in quantitative angiography. Am J Cardiol 1991;68(11):1176–82.

63. Mauri L, O'Malley AJ, Popma JJ, et al. Comparison of thrombosis and restenosis risk from stent length of sirolimus-eluting stents versus bare metal stents. Am J Cardiol 2005;95(10):1140–5.

64. Stone GW, Reifart NJ, Moussa I, et al. Percutaneous recanalization of chronically occluded coronary arteries: a consensus document: part II. Circulation 2005;112(16):2530–7.

65. Stone GW, Kandzari DE, Mehran R, et al. Percutaneous recanalization of chronically occluded coronary arteries: a consensus document: part I. Circulation 2005;112(15):2364–72.

66. Dvir D, Assali A, Kornowski R. Percutaneous coronary intervention for chronic total occlusion: novel 3-dimensional imaging and quantitative analysis. Catheter Cardiovasc Interv 2008;71(6):784–9.

67. Ramcharitar S, Patterson MS, van Geuns RJ, et al. Magnetic navigation system used successfully to cross a crushed stent in a bifurcation that failed with conventional wires. Catheter Cardiovasc Interv 2007;69(6):852–5.

68. Tsuchida K, García-García H, Tanimoto S, et al. Feasibility and safety of guidewire navigation using a magnetic navigation system in coronary artery stenoses. EuroInterv 2005;1:329–35.

69. Coles DR, Smail MA, Negus IS, et al. Comparison of radiation doses from multislice computed tomography coronary angiography and conventional diagnostic angiography. J Am Coll Cardiol 2006;47(9):1840–5.

70. Dill T, Deetjen A, Ekinci O, et al. Radiation dose exposure in multislice computed tomography of the coronaries in comparison with conventional coronary angiography. Int J Cardiol 2008;124(3):307–11.

71. Jabara R, Chronos N, Klein L, et al. Comparison of multidetector 64-slice computed tomographic angiography to coronary angiography to assess the patency of coronary artery bypass grafts. Am J Cardiol 2007;99(11):1529–34.

72. Slager CJ, Wentzel JJ, Schuurbiers JC, et al. True 3-dimensional reconstruction of coronary arteries in patients by fusion of angiography and IVUS (ANGUS) and its quantitative validation. Circulation 2000;102(5):511–6.

73. Chen SJ, Carroll JD. 3-D reconstruction of coronary arterial tree to optimize angiographic visualization. IEEE Trans Med Imaging 2000;19(4):318–36.

74. Messenger JC, Chen SJ, Carroll JD, et al. 3D coronary reconstruction from routine single-plane coronary angiograms: clinical validation and quantitative analysis of the right coronary artery in 100 patients. Int J Card Imaging 2000;16(6):413–27.

75. Feldman CL, Stone PH. Intravascular hemodynamic factors responsible for progression of coronary atherosclerosis and development of vulnerable plaque. Curr Opin Cardiol 2000;15(6):430–40.

76. Katritsis DG, Pantos J, Efstathopoulos E. Hemodynamic factors and atheromatic plaque rupture in the coronary arteries: from vulnerable plaque to vulnerable coronary segment. Coron Artery Dis 2007;18(3):229–37.

77. Katritsis D, Kaiktsis L, Chaniotis A, et al. Wall shear stress: theoretical considerations and methods of measurement. Prog Cardiovasc Dis 2007;49(5):307–29.

78. Soulis JV, Giannoglou GD, Parcharidis GE, et al. Flow parameters in normal left coronary artery tree. Implication to atherogenesis. Comput Biol Med 2007;37(5):628–36.

79. Johnston BM, Johnston PR, Corney S, et al. Non-newtonian blood flow in human right coronary arteries: transient simulations. J Biomech 2006;39(6):1116–28.

80. Wentzel JJ, Gijsen FJ, Stergiopulos N, et al. Shear stress, vascular remodeling and neointimal formation. J Biomech 2003;36(5):681–8.

Computer Assistance for Solving Imaging Problems

Joel A. Garcia, MD[a,b,]*, Babak Movassaghi, PhD[c]

KEYWORDS

- Computer assistance • Angiography • Coronary
- Rotational angiography • Foreshortening • Overlap
- Optimal view map • Universal view map

Imaging artifacts inherent in two-dimensional (2D) projection of complex three-dimensional (3D) structures in standard angiography limit its usefulness in making vascular evaluations.[1,2] Innovative 3D reconstruction software based on CT, magnetic resonance (MR), and planar imaging are major advances in the diagnosis and treatment of endovascular diseases. With the use of advance processing, these imaging techniques provide 3D vessel evaluations and characteristics that have important clinical implications. Meanwhile, standard angiography, while a well-established technique, has not been so readily used to provide 3D reconstructions because of imaging artifacts inherent in two-dimensional (2D) projection of complex 3D structures.[1,2] Now, though, computers can be used to correct most of these known inaccuracies in x-ray based angiography.[3–7] Furthermore, a computer-based technique applied in standard angiography can precisely characterize stent-induced conformational changes in three dimensions.[8–12]

In determining the risk associated with a given lesion, it is necessary to measure such vessel properties as tortuosity, length, and take-off angles, and to determine bifurcation and ostium characteristics.[13] These properties and characteristics are best evaluated in 3D representations of the vascular tree. For this reason, images showing dynamic conformational changes of the vascular tree should also play a role in the treatment planning process.

Two-dimensional imaging techniques can also be used to represent and measure these variables. However, the accuracy of such representations and measurements is often limited.[1,14] These 2D techniques of image acquisition with traditional angiography are nonstandardized, subjectively chosen, and are highly dependent upon the 3D visual skills of individual operators.[4] By contrast, a 3D evaluation of a vessel yields an accurate representation of clinically relevant vessel properties and characteristics and incorporates important dynamic changes.[8,12,15–20] Three-dimensional quantification of these changes eliminates dependence on the user's visual estimation and standardizes the vessel-evaluation process, therefore minimizing inaccuracies. Contemporary medicine has evolved along with imaging techniques. The traditional 2D planar imaging evaluation is now complemented by biplane angiography, rotational angiography, CT, and MR. Some of these widely used techniques, such as CT and MR, already are used in making 3D vascular evaluations.[21–38]

In an era of complex and expensive interventions with drug-eluting stents and other devices, precise length measurements and accurate

a Medicine Department, Division of Cardiology, University of Colorado at Denver, 12401 E 17th Ave, Box B-132 Leprino Building, Rm 524, Aurora, CO 80045, USA
b Medicine Department, Division of Cardiology, Denver Health Medical Center, 777 Bannock street, MC 0960, Denver, CO 80204, USA
c Philips Healthcare, Research Department, 12401 E 17th Ave, Box B-132 Leprino Building, Rm 524, Aurora, CO 80045, USA
* Corresponding author. Denver Health Medical Center (DHMC), University of Colorado Hospital at Denver and Health Sciences Center (UCDHSC), 777 Bannock Street, Mail Code 0960, Denver, CO 80204.
E-mail address: joel.garcia@dhha.org (J.A. Garcia).

Cardiol Clin 27 (2009) 503–512
doi:10.1016/j.ccl.2009.03.009
0733-8651/09/$ – see front matter © 2009 Elsevier Inc. All rights reserved.

placement are critical to minimize the need for additional interventions resulting from inaccurate or incomplete imaging. Recognition of these limitations has resulted in the development of imaging techniques designed to specifically address the weaknesses of the traditional angiographic approach.[8,9,16,19,39–46] Advanced computer-assisted technologies capable of minimizing the shortcomings of traditional angiography have been developed and are now in clinical use.

CURRENT ANGIOGRAPHIC TECHNIQUES

The placement of the gantry in a location to produce useful angiographic information is a fundamental task in both diagnostic imaging but also in the performance of endovascular interventions. Obtaining optimal angiographic views is critical to assessing lesion morphology, extent of disease, and involvement of major branch segments.[14] These considerations have become more prominent since the advent of interventional cardiology because, with interventional cardiology, the precision is more important and evaluation goes beyond simply noting the quality of distal conduits for bypass surgery.

Three-dimensional vascular trees registered or aligned in the coordinate system of gantry location can be used to perform the imaging tasks commonly encountered. First, overlap of vessels in the tree needs to be minimized. Second, segments of the tree need to be imaged with the imaging system perpendicular to the axis of the vessel segment such that no foreshortening is produced in the resultant projection image. Third, the specific bifurcation points need to be accurately imaged.

Coronary Modeling

The 3D modeling technique uses 3D centerline data and shaded or rendered surfaces; the diameter and 3D morphologic structure of the vessel is subsequently derived with a computer algorithm. This 3D "modeling" technique uses two or more angiographic projections to extract features of the vessel and create a 3D representation. Modeling can be obtained on line and off line from various imaging modalities. It can be obtained from standard angiography, rotational angiography, and extended acquisitions.

Coronary Reconstruction

Several methods capable of generating 3D images have been described and, in general, can be classified as either surface-rendering techniques or volume-rendering techniques.

Three-dimensional reconstruction images can be generated from techniques that acquire volumetric data points. These techniques include rotational angiography, CT, and MRI. The surface-rendering method relies upon a computer algorithm to reconstruct intensity values. The resultant image is a representation of the surface contour and appears 3D through computer-generated shading. The maximum intensity projection algorithm is another commonly used surface-rendering technique.

Volume rendering uses all the data and reconstructs all data points without shading or computer enhancement.

FORESHORTENING, OVERLAP, AND BIFURCATION LESIONS

Vessel foreshortening and overlap are recognized imaging artifacts that result from the 2D angiographic projection of 3D vascular structures.[1,2] The tortuosity of coronary artery segments present specific challenges in minimizing vessel foreshortening and angiographically separating adjacent structures.

The clinical implications of unrecognized foreshortening include missed lesions, errors in assessing lesion length, incomplete coverage of lesions by stents, underestimation of stenosis severity, and inaccurate quantitative coronary angiography calculations.

Vessel overlap, a result of one vessel or segment superimposed on another, prevents complete image interpretation. As opposed to vessel foreshortening, vessel overlap is easily recognized by the operator and does not require significant image processing.

Ostial lesions are traditionally difficult to image because of challenges in avoiding the ostium of the vessel to be covered by the main branch or a contiguous vessel. Screening angiographic evaluations are often limited in providing a complete ostial vessel survey, thus requiring multiple subsequent angiograms.

THE NEED FOR COMPUTER ASSISTANCE IN DETERMINING OPTIMAL VIEWS

Sometimes even experienced intervenionalists fail to choose the best view for minimizing image foreshortening of the diseased segment,[14,41] even though several methods are readily available to produce useful images that avoid overlap and minimize foreshortening for all segments of interest in the vascular tree.[3,39–41]

Computer graphics can be used to display the tree in a variety of views (3D modeling and 3D reconstruction) and the operator can select appropriate views (**Fig. 1**). Alternatively algorithms can be written to automatically process the data, recommend specific views, or produce visual guides that combine a parameter, such as the extent of foreshortening for a vessel segment of interest, for all possible angiographic views. The later approach is represented by a color-coded map of the degree of foreshortening and overlap for all possible gantry locations (**Fig. 2**).

PATIENT-SPECIFIC OPTIMAL VIEW MAP

Three-dimensional vascular trees generated with CT angiography, MR angiography, or traditional x-ray technology can be used to simulate all possible angiographic views of the vascular tree. The principle that 3D data sets can be used to simulate 2D images is an important practical approach needed in endovascular interventions since the image-guidance of multiple techniques remains to be fluoroscopy. With the expanded use of CT angiography and MR angiography, making the best use of information from each diagnostic modality when the patient comes to interventional therapy is increasingly important.

The clinical value of using a 3D vascular tree to simulate angiographic views is to enhance patient safety and potentially improve interventional outcomes. Computer computation of an optimal view can be done before the intervention as part of the planning process for the procedure. For the interventional procedures, the traditional trial-and-error method of finding good angiographic

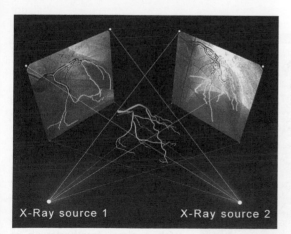

X-Ray source 1   X-Ray source 2

Fig. 1. Three-dimensional modeling concept. Two orthogonal views result in the forward projection of a computer-generated image. (*Adapted from* Garcia JA, Movassaghi B, Casserly IP, et al. Determination of optimal viewing regions for x-ray coronary angiography based on a quantitative analysis of 3D reconstructed models. Int J Cardiovasc Imaging 2009;25:455–62; with permission.)

views is often costly in expending time, radiation, and contrast. Optimizing working views for interventions theoretically should reduce visualization-related mistakes and prevent complications. Several groups have demonstrated the value of using a 3D vascular tree to simulate angiographic views.[5,6,47–49]

How is the Optimal View Map Created?

With the use of a rotational acquisition protocol (cranial or caudal), with any field of view, a 3D modeling of the left coronary artery (LCA) system is completed. The reconstruction is performed with the use of 3D modeling software commercially available via various vendors.

Once the rotational run is completed, it is transferred to a dedicated 3D workstation where the analysis is performed. Current systems automatically transfer the image sequence to the workstation for modeling/reconstruction in under 60 seconds. The system is designed to generate a complete model of the artery after various steps. First, the operator must identify two orthogonal views of the target coronary tree. Second, both views should be completely or partially gated to the ECG. This step is not mandatory for modeling, but ensures greater precision. Third, points in the vascular tree must be recognized by clicking on them on both views. The generation of a computer-created 3D model follows. The results provide three important clinical results: (1) a 3D model that enables measurements of length and size, (2) an optimal view map, and (3) the gantry position of all intended views in the optimal view map (**Fig. 3**).

How is the Optimal View Map Used?

Using the modeled/reconstructed images obtained from the workstation, the best working view and lesion length can be identified with no extra contrast or fluoroscopy/cine use. The 3D-assisted best working view represents the least foreshortening. This avoids underestimation of the severity of the lesion, avoids treatment of side branches, and identifies the accurate length needed for stent selection (see **Fig. 3**). The current Phillips FD-20 system (Philips Healthcare, Best, The Netherlands), which generated the images for this article, is one of several imaging systems capable of automatically setting itself to the best working view.

UNIVERSAL OPTIMAL VIEW MAP

Using previously validated 3D modeling techniques in a large patient cohort undergoing coronary angiography, a recent study identified

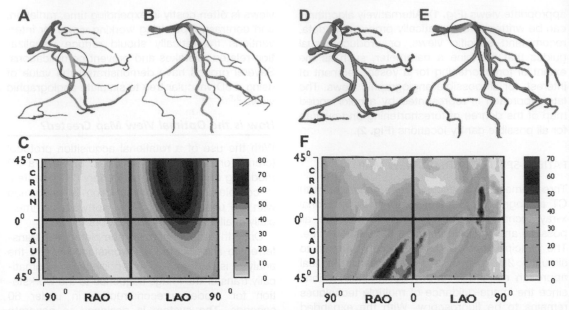

Fig. 2. Generation of segment-specific optimal view map. (*A* and *B*) Two projection views of modeled left coronary artery corresponding to the overlap optimal view map (*C*) of the vessel segment shown as a green centerline in *A* and *B*. Projection image *A* corresponds to a yellow region and projection image *B* to a red region in the optimal view map (*C*) where yellow regions illustrate minimum vessel overlap and red regions illustrate severe vessel overlap. Similarly, 2d and 2e show two projection views of modeled left coronary artery corresponding to the overlap optimal view map (*2f*) of the vessel segment shown as a green centerline in 2d and 2e. CAUD, caudal; CRAN, cranial; LAO, left anterior oblique; RAO, right anterior oblique.

optimal view regions for first- and second-order coronary segments that minimized vessel foreshortening and overlap with the goal of reducing imaging inaccuracies. Within the viewing regions identified, the minimum vessel foreshortening was 5.8% ± 3.9% for the left coronary artery and

5.6% ± 3.6% for the right coronary artery, and the average overlap was 8.7% ± 7.9% for the left coronary artery and 4.6% ± 3.2% for the right coronary artery. This represents the first scientific validation of optimal viewing regions to guide diagnostic and interventional coronary procedures.[41]

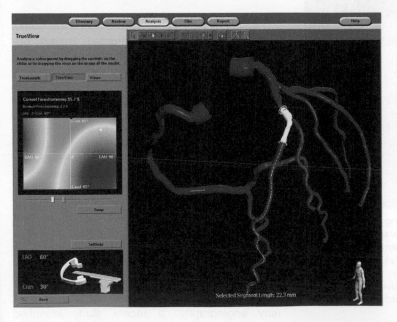

Fig. 3. Three-dimensional modeling/reconstruction station. The coronary model allows for size and length evaluations, the optimal view map (*color coded*), and the gantry position. This example shows on the coronary model how the mid–left anterior descending artery highlighted segment measures 22.3 mm. The optimal view map shows a white point (LAO 60°–Cran 30°) where there is 15.7% foreshortening. The black point represents a computer-suggested gantry with minimal foreshortening at 1.2%. Finally, the gantry shows its position at LAO 60°–Cran 30° in the left lower corner. Caud, caudal; Cran, cranial; LAO, left anterior oblique; RAO, right anterior oblique.

In general, the optimal viewing regions for individual coronary segments defined in this study match viewing angles previously recommended by experts. However, there are some notable exceptions: the right anterior oblique cranial region proved optimal for viewing the mid–left anterior descending artery, the posteroanterior caudal region for viewing the proximal left main, and right anterior oblique caudal region for viewing the mid posterior descending artery.[41]

For current interventional procedures, where decisions regarding device length may be hampered by failure to appreciate vessel foreshortening, the optimal viewing regions defined in the mentioned study may provide important scientifically based guidance that could be especially useful in laboratories where 3D modeling and patient-specific optimal view maps are currently unavailable.

While we have sought to validate optimal viewing regions applicable to a broad population undergoing coronary angiography, we believe that the future will be dominated by a patient-specific approach that will deliver superior results (**Fig. 4**).

NEW IMAGING TRAJECTORIES

New x-ray systems are now capable of acquiring trajectories where the C-arm moves freely around the patient while capturing data. With the incorporation of the universal optimal view map, investigators are now able to design new imaging trajectories that can cover all required gantries for a complete diagnostic evaluation in a single sweep.

These imaging trajectories aim at covering all spots in the view map that minimize foreshortening and overlap for each coronary segment (**Fig. 5**). A study is currently investigating the feasibility and clinical impact of these trajectories compared with standard angiography.

DATABASE CREATION

The generation of 3D vascular data on large numbers of patients undergoing diagnostic imaging with CT angiography, MR angiography, or 3D processed angiographic images provides an opportunity to catalog anatomical features in the form of databases. Subsequent evaluation

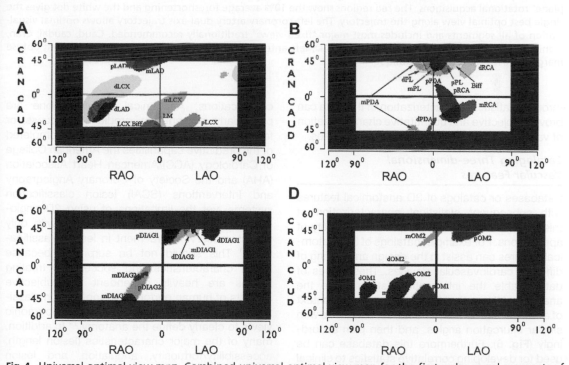

Fig. 4. Universal optimal view map. Combined universal optimal view map for the first-order vessel segments of the left coronary artery (*A*) and right coronary artery (RCA) (*B*). Combined universal optimal view map of the second-order vessel segments of the left coronary artery (*C*, *D*). Biff, bifurcation; CAUD, caudal; CRAN, cranial; d, distal; DIAG, diagonal; LAD, left anterior descending artery; LAO, left anterior oblique; LCX, left circumflex artery; LM, left main; m, mid; OM, obtuse marginal; p, proximal; PDA, posterior descending artery; PL, postero-lateral; RAO, right anterior oblique. (*Adapted from* Garcia JA, Movassaghi B, Casserly IP, et al. Determination of optimal viewing regions for x-ray coronary angiography based on a quantitative analysis of 3D reconstructed models. Int J Cardiovasc Imaging 2009;25:455–62; with permission.)

	Proximal	**Mid**	**Distal**

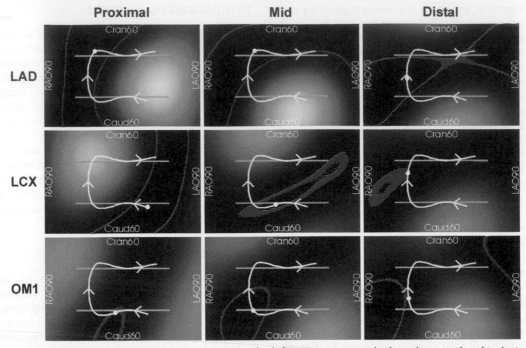

Fig. 5. The development of new imaging trajectories. The left coronary artery dual-motion rotational trajectory is shown in yellow on each individual vessel segment average optimal view map. The green lines show the two "in plane" rotational acquisitions. The red regions show the 10% average foreshortening and the white dot gives the single best optimal view along the trajectory. The left coronary artery dual-axis trajectory allows optimal visualization of all segments and includes most major "fixed views" traditionally recommended. Caud, caudal; Cran, cranial; LAD, left anterior descending artery; LAO, left anterior oblique; LCX, left circumflex; OM1, first obtuse marginal; RAO, right anterior oblique.

through statistical characterization of this data can provide objective and quantitative characterization of vascular anatomy serving different purposes.

Cataloging Three-dimensional Vascular Features

Databases or catalogs of 3D anatomical features with subsequent statistical characterization of this human in vivo data are useful for a variety of applications. For example, catalogs of 3D anatomical features can assist in the design and testing of different cardiovascular devices. These types of data enable the interventionalist to place the anatomy of the patient being treated in the context of anatomies of similar patients, such as those with similar bifurcation angles, and then plan accordingly (**Fig. 6**). Furthermore this database can be used for developing correlative statistics to clinical outcomes of interventions.

Traditional lesion classification systems have been using 2D angiographic images and have been shown to be useful in predicting the outcome of coronary interventions and the need to use adjunctive devices.[13] Clinical features combined with these anatomical features can predict

complications. Anatomical features alone are particularly powerful in predicting success or failure. Validation studies have been completed of the predictive capabilities the American College of Cardiology (ACC)/American Heart Association (AHA) and the Society of Coronary Angiography and Interventions (SCAI) lesion classification systems, yet the limitations of using 2D angiographic data also have been defined with only fair interobserver agreement in lesion classification.[13] This should not be surprising because lesion characteristics and success in treating lesions are heavily dependent on subjective aspects of human performance not only in classifying lesions but in acquiring suitable angiographic views to clearly define the anatomy.[14] In addition, many of the major characteristics (lesion length, accessibility/tortuosity, angulation, and lesion eccentricity) may be misrepresented and poorly quantified in 2D projection images because of foreshortening, overlap, and other limitations of traditional angiography. As pointed out in the recently released percutaneous coronary intervention guidelines, no prospective studies using core laboratory analysis have validated systems of

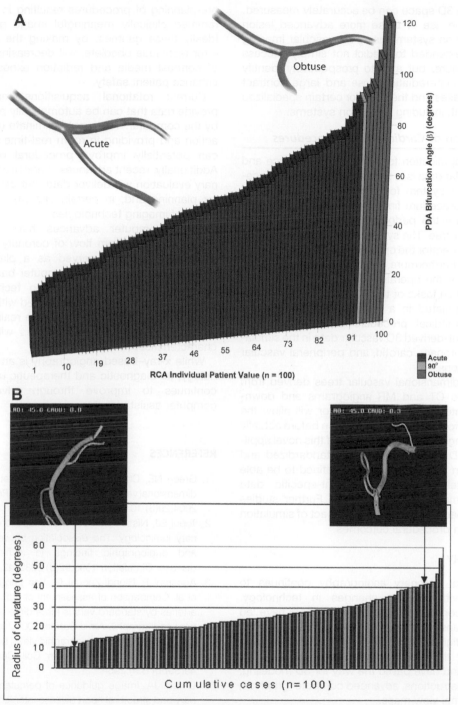

Fig. 6. (*A*) Posterior descending artery (PDA) bifurcation angle database. Note the variation in angle behavior in these 100 right coronary artery–posterior descending artery bifurcations. The spectrum of angles goes from acute to obtuse. (*B*) Right coronary artery curvature database. This is the spectrum of radius of curvature in 100 right coronary arteries. The spectrum of curvature goes from 0° to 55°.

lesion and target-vessel classification to stratify the risk of success and complications.

Alternatively more elaborate, sophisticated, objective, and standardized lesion classification systems can be designed and tested for predictive value for interventional outcomes using 3D computer assistance. For example, tortuosity can be measured in units of curvature/torsion and lengths in 3D space can be accurately measured. Finally, the use of these more advanced lesion classification systems using 3D vascular imaging may be extended to predict not simply success versus failure, but also to prospectively identify the long high-radiation dose and large contract volume cases and the need for certain specialized equipment, including navigation systems.

Simulation of Cardiovascular Procedures

Another application for computer assistance and 3D vascular data is in simulation of medical procedures.[50] A system for simulating a fluoroscopic medical procedure first must enable an operator to simulate the performance of a procedure in a vascular tree. The system should also, however, give the operator the option of selecting any gantry position. Furthermore, the 3D vascular trees are needed for the operator to master the hand-eye coordination tasks of the interventional technique being simulated in a realistic vascular system. Current medical procedure simulators already use patient-derived 3D vascular data in the simulation of coronary, carotid, and peripheral vascular interventions.

Three-dimensional vascular trees derived from diagnostic CT and MR angiograms and downloaded into a procedure simulator will allow the operator to practice an intervention before actually performing it. To make the most of this novel application, 3D data files must be standardized and simulation technology must be refined to be able immediately incorporate patient-specific data into a simulated case structure. Further studies will be needed to evaluate the impact of simulation training in procedural outcomes.

SUMMARY

Traditional coronary angiography continues to evolve with ongoing changes in technology. Current computer-based advancements have led to the transformation of cine-based acquisitions into all-digital formats. These all-digital formats allow for the advanced processing of acquired images and have paved the way for 3D modeling, 3D reconstructions, advanced computer graphics, and optimal view maps.

Three-dimensional modeling has been well described and provides the basis for a fast in-room evaluation, which, coupled with optimal view maps, aims at minimizing imaging inaccuracies while providing a superior safety profile through less exposure to radiation and contrast.[3,4,39,41]

Universal and, most importantly, patient-specific optimal view maps will allow for the pre-planning of procedures resulting in preprogrammed clinically meaningful image gantries.[41] Ideally these gantries, by making the trial-and-error technique obsolete, will decreasing the use of contrast media and radiation exposure thus enhance patient safety.

Current rotational acquisitions may soon provide data that can be automatically processed by the computer. This would eliminate user interaction and providing in-room real-time data that can potentially improve procedural outcomes. Additionally, recent advances in noninvasive coronary evaluation will deliver data that can be used for planning and, in certain circumstances, the fusion of imaging technologies.

These computer advances have not only improved the in-room flow of coronary interventions but have also served as a platform for medical education through computer-based simulations.[50] Data from all imaging technologies, collected in a database and coupled with medical simulation, can form the basis of a realistic environment for practicing procedures with similar characteristics.[50]

While x-ray–based angiography is an old technology, its diagnostic and therapeutic usefulness continues to improve through advances in computer assistance.

REFERENCES

1. Green NE, Chen SY, Messenger JC, et al. Three-dimensional vascular angiography. Curr Probl Cardiol 2004;29(3):104–42.
2. Topol EJ, Nissen SE. Our preoccupation with coronary luminology. The dissociation between clinical and angiographic findings in ischemic heart disease. Circulation 1995;92(8):2333–42.
3. Agostoni P, Biondi-Zoccai G, Van Langenhove G, et al. Comparison of assessment of native coronary arteries by standard versus three-dimensional coronary angiography. Am J Cardiol 2008;102(3):272–9.
4. Garcia JA. Optimal angiographic views based on 3D reconstructed models. J Am Coll Cardiol 2007; 49(Suppl B:9):296A.
5. Garcia JA. Image guidance of percutaneous coronary and structural heart disease interventions using a CT and fluoroscopy integration. Vascular Disease Management 2007;4(3):1–4.
6. Garcia JA, Bhakta S, Kay J, et al. On-line multi-slice computed tomography interactive overlay with conventional x-ray: a new and advanced imaging fusion concept. Int J Cardiol 2009;133(3):e101–5. Epub Jan 29, 2008.
7. Garcia JA, Chen J, Hansgen A, et al. Rotational angiography (RA) and three-dimensional imaging

(3-DRA): an available clinical tool. Int J Cardiovasc Imaging 2007;23(1):9–13.

8. Chen SJ, Carroll JD. 3-D reconstruction of coronary arterial tree to optimize angiographic visualization. IEEE Trans Med Imaging 2000;19(4):318–36.

9. Chen SJ, Hoffmann KR, Carroll JD. Three-dimensional reconstruction of coronary arterial tree based on biplane angiograms. SPIE. Medical Imaging. 1996;2710:103–14.

10. Chen SY, Carroll JD. Kinematic and deformation analysis of 4-D coronary arterial trees reconstructed from cine angiograms. IEEE Trans Med Imaging 2003;22(6):710–21.

11. Chen SY, Carroll JD, Messenger JC. Quantitative analysis of reconstructed 3-D coronary arterial tree and intracoronary devices. IEEE Trans Med Imaging 2002;21(7):724–40.

12. Messenger JC, Chen SY, Carroll JD, et al. 3D coronary reconstruction from routine single-plane coronary angiograms: clinical validation and quantitative analysis of the right coronary artery in 100 patients. Int J Card Imaging 2000;16(6):413–27.

13. Scanlon PJ, Faxon DP, Audet AM, et al. ACC/AHA guidelines for coronary angiography. A report of the American College of Cardiology/American Heart Association Task Force on practice guidelines (Committee on Coronary Angiography). Developed in collaboration with the Society for Cardiac Angiography and Interventions. J Am Coll Cardiol 1999; 33(6):1756–824.

14. Green NE, Chen SY, Hansgen AR, et al. Angiographic views used for percutaneous coronary interventions: a three-dimensional analysis of physician-determined vs. computer-generated views. Catheter Cardiovasc Interv 2005;64(4):451–9.

15. Chen SY, Metz CE. Improved determination of biplane imaging geometry from two projection images and its application to three-dimensional reconstruction of coronary arterial trees. Med Phys 1997;24(5):633–54.

16. Ding Z, Friedman MH. Quantification of 3-D coronary arterial motion using clinical biplane cineangiograms. Int J Card Imaging 2000;16(5):331–46.

17. Gross MF, Friedman MH. Dynamics of coronary artery curvature obtained from biplane cineangiograms. J Biomech 1998;31(5):479–84.

18. Hoffmann KR, Metz CE, Chen Y. Determination of 3D imaging geometry and object configurations from two biplane views: an enhancement of the Metz-Fencil technique. Med Phys 1995;22(8): 1219–27.

19. Movassaghi B, Rasche V, Grass M, et al. A quantitative analysis of 3-D coronary modeling from two or more projection images. IEEE Trans Med Imaging 2004;23(12):1517–31.

20. Shechter G, Devernay F, Coste-Maniere E, et al. Three-dimensional motion tracking of coronary arteries in biplane cineangiograms. IEEE Trans Med Imaging 2003;22(4):493–503.

21. Becker A, Leber A, White CW, et al. Multislice computed tomography for determination of coronary artery disease in a symptomatic patient population. Int J Cardiovasc Imaging 2007;23(3):361–7. Epub Dec 8, 2006.

22. Budoff MJ. Noninvasive coronary angiography using computed tomography. Expert Rev Cardiovasc Ther 2005;3(1):123–32.

23. Budoff MJ, Gopal A, Gul KM, et al. Prevalence of obstructive coronary artery disease in an outpatient cardiac CT angiography environment. Int J Cardiol 2008;129(1):32–6.

24. Budoff MJ, Rasouli ML, Shavelle DM, et al. Cardiac CT angiography (CTA) and nuclear myocardial perfusion imaging (MPI)—a comparison in detecting significant coronary artery disease. Acad Radiol 2007;14(3):252–7.

25. de Feyter P, Mollet NR, Cadermartiri F, et al. MS-CT coronary imaging. J Interv Cardiol 2003;16(6):465–8.

26. Gaemperli O, Schepis T, Koepfli P, et al. Accuracy of 64-slice CT angiography for the detection of functionally relevant coronary stenoses as assessed with myocardial perfusion SPECT. Eur J Nucl Med Mol Imaging 2007;34(8):1162–71. Epub Jan 12, 2007.

27. Johnson TR, Nikolaou K, Wintersperger BJ, et al. Dual-source CT cardiac imaging: initial experience. Eur Radiol 2006;16(7):1409–15. Epub May 13, 2006.

28. Langerak SE, Vliegen HW, Jukema JW, et al. Value of magnetic resonance imaging for the noninvasive detection of stenosis in coronary artery bypass grafts and recipient coronary arteries. Circulation 2003;107(11):1502–8.

29. Langreck H, Schnackenburg B, Nehrke K, et al. MR coronary artery imaging with 3D motion adapted gating (MAG) in comparison to a standard prospective navigator technique. J Cardiovasc Magn Reson 2005;7(5):793–7.

30. Leber AW, Becker A, Knez A, et al. Accuracy of 64-slice computed tomography to classify and quantify plaque volumes in the proximal coronary system: a comparative study using intravascular ultrasound. J Am Coll Cardiol 2006;47(3):672–7.

31. Leber AW, Knez A, Becker A, et al. Visualising non-calcified coronary plaques by CT. Int J Cardiovasc Imaging 2005;21(1):55–61.

32. Leschka S, Alkadhi H, Plass A, et al. Accuracy of MSCT coronary angiography with 64-slice technology: first experience. Eur Heart J 2005;26(15): 1482–7.

33. Manning WJ, Nezafat R, Appelbaum E, et al. Coronary magnetic resonance imaging. Magn Reson Imaging Clin N Am 2007;15(4):609–37, vii.

34. Nikolaou K, Knez A, Rist C, et al. Accuracy of 64-MDCT in the diagnosis of ischemic heart disease. AJR Am J Roentgenol 2006;187(1):111–7.

35. Paulin S, von Schulthess GK, Fossel E, et al. MR imaging of the aortic root and proximal coronary arteries. AJR Am J Roentgenol 1987;148(4):665–70.

36. Sakuma H. [Cardiac MRI: current status and future prospective]. Nippon Igaku Hoshasen Gakkai Zasshi 2003;63(1):21–5 [in Japanese].

37. Sakuma H [Cardiac magnetic resonance imaging]. Kyobu Geka 2007;60(8 Suppl):635–41 [in Japanese].

38. Sakuma H, Goto M, Nomura Y, et al. Three-dimensional coronary magnetic resonance angiography with injection of extracellular contrast medium. Invest Radiol 1999;34(8):503–8.

39. Garcia JA, Chen J, Hansgen A, et al. Rotational angiography (RA) and three-dimensional imaging (3-DRA): an available clinical tool. Int J Cardiovasc Imaging 2007;23(1):9–13. Epub Jun 16, 2006.

40. Garcia JA, Chen SY, Messenger JC, et al. Initial clinical experience of selective coronary angiography using one prolonged injection and a 180 degrees rotational trajectory. Catheter Cardiovasc Interv 2007 Aug 1;70(2):190–6.

41. Garcia JA, Movassaghi B, Casserly IP, et al. Determination of optimal viewing regions for x-ray coronary angiography based on a quantitative analysis of 3D reconstructed models. Int J Cardiovasc Imaging 2008 Dec 20 [Epub ahead of print].

42. Gollapudi RR, Valencia R, Lee SS, et al. Utility of three-dimensional reconstruction of coronary angiography to guide percutaneous coronary intervention. Catheter Cardiovasc Interv 2007;69(4):479–82.

43. Gradaus R, Mathies K, Breithardt G, et al. Clinical assessment of a new real time 3D quantitative coronary angiography system: evaluation in stented vessel segments. Catheter Cardiovasc Interv 2006;68(1):44–9.

44. Movassaghi B, Schaefer D, Grass M, et al. 3D reconstruction of coronary stents in vivo based on motion compensated x-ray angiograms. Med Image Comput Comput Assist Interv Int Conf Med Image Comput Comput Assist Interv 2006;9(Pt 2):177–84.

45. Rasche V, Buecker A, Grass M, et al. ECG-gated 3D-rotational coronary angiography (3DRCA). Paris (France): Springer; 2002.

46. Rasche V, Movassaghi B, Grass M, et al. Automatic selection of the optimal cardiac phase for gated three-dimensional coronary x-ray angiography. Acad Radiol 2006;13(5):630–40.

47. Budoff MJ, Gopal A, Gopalakrishnan D. Cardiac computed tomography: diagnostic utility and integration in clinical practice. Clin Cardiol 2006;29(9 Suppl 1):I4–I14.

48. de Feyter PJ, Nieman K. New coronary imaging techniques: what to expect? Heart 2002;87(3):195–7.

49. Hecht HS. Applications of multislice coronary computed tomographic angiography to percutaneous coronary intervention: How did we ever do without it? Catheter Cardiovasc Interv 2008;71(4):490–503.

50. Carroll JD, Messenger JC. Medical simulation: the new tool for training and skill assessment. Perspect Biol Med 2008;51(1):47–60.

Coronary Computed Tomographic Angiography in the Cardiac Catheterization Laboratory: Current Applications and Future Developments

Onno Wink, PhD[a],*, Harvey S. Hecht, MD[b],
Daniel Ruijters, MSc[c]

KEYWORDS

- CTA • PCI • Coronary interventions
- Coronary angiography • Roadmapping

The last few years have seen a marked increase in the number of cardiac CT scans performed, regardless of reimbursement issues and concerns about radiation dose. New generation multidetector CT (MDCT) scanners with wide craniocaudal coverage (256 slices and beyond) have the potential to further improve the diagnostic capability compared with that of the existing generation of MDCT scanners. In addition, new dose-reduction technologies are now available on these scanners, making it possible to provide high-quality coronary imaging with a significant reduction in radiation dose. Although single- and multicenter diagnostic accuracy studies of coronary CT angiography (CCTA) using existing technology (16–64 slices) have demonstrated MDCT's capability in ruling out coronary artery disease (CAD) with negative predictive values greater than 96%,[1–7] the ability to precisely define CAD has varied, leading to the common perception that CCTA cannot adequately deal with complex CAD.[8] Recent advances, and the appropriate use of commonly available analytic tools, permit the extraction of the remarkable data offered by this technology and show its potential to have an impact on planning catheter coronary angiography (CCA) and percutaneous coronary intervention (PCI) performed in the cardiac catheterization laboratory.

ADVANCES IN CORONARY CT ANGIOGRAPHY ACQUISITIONS

Current CT scanners provide increased coverage (8–16 cm/rotation) and shorter acquisition times. The newer 256-slice (Brilliance iCT, Philips Healthcare) and 320-slice (Aquilion One, Toshiba Medical Systems) MDCT scanners decrease the likelihood of patient motion, respiration, and heart rate variations that degrade image quality.[9] In addition, improved temporal resolution is associated with

[a] Philips Healthcare, Cardio/Vascular X-ray, Leprino Building Room 501, 12401 East 17th Avenue, Aurora, CO 80045, USA
[b] Department of Interventional Cardiology, Lenox Hill Hospital, 9th Floor, 130 East 77th Street, New York, NY, 10021, USA
[c] Philips Healthcare, Cardio/Vascular Innovation, Veenpluis 6, Building QJ2116, 5680DA Best, The Netherlands
* Corresponding author.
E-mail address: onno.wink@philips.com (O. Wink).

Cardiol Clin 27 (2009) 513–529
doi:10.1016/j.ccl.2009.04.002

faster rotation speeds (Brilliance iCT) and dual-source technology (Somatom Definition, Siemens Healthcare), minimizing artifacts arising from cardiac motion. Improvements on detector technology (Discovery CT750 HD, GE Healthcare) are expected to result in better spatial resolution. Another area currently being investigated is dual-energy imaging, aimed to minimize the blooming effects of thick calcification or potentially allow for a distinction between types of plaque. In addition to this continuous development in the scanner technology, smarter acquisition techniques and improved injection protocols have dramatically reduced the amount of radiation while providing images of superior quality. As an example, prospectively gated axial imaging for CCTA (or "step and shoot"), with radiation applied only during the middiastolic coronary rest phase, has demonstrated radiation dose savings of greater than 75% compared with the traditional technique of helical retrospective gating while maintaining image quality,[10–14] and with a diagnostic accuracy greater than 96%.[15,16] By combining more intelligent acquisition protocols and improved hardware capabilities, some manufacturers predict a complete diagnostic study with less than 2 mSv in the not-too-distant future.

REVIEWING CORONARY CT ANGIOGRAPHY

After reconstruction, the CTA volume is sent to a digital workstation for further processing and to allow detailed analysis of the coronary arteries. This section details common segmentation and extraction techniques of the areas of interest from the CT datasets, and discusses different visualization techniques that can be used to aid the reviewer in arriving at a proper diagnosis and an appropriate assessment of the extent of the patient's coronary disease.

Basic Reviewing Tools

By stacking up the unprocessed (or raw) two-dimensional (2D) CT images, the three-dimensional (3D) data set is formed and consists of volume elements or voxels. Each voxel's intensity is based on its corresponding Hounsfield unit (HU), reflecting its radiopacity. Routine review of the CT data by browsing through the axial images (consisting of only one layer of voxels) allows for a quick scan for potential disease, but does not allow for sophisticated data segmentation or extraction. The next step for the user is to freely define a set of cross-sectional planes that cut through the CT volume with a slab thickness that can be varied. Within the slab, generally the

maximum intensity projection technique is used to display the brightest voxels. The operator has the freedom to create multiple oblique rotations of these slabs. The latter technique is the most common analytic method, primarily because it requires virtually no postprocessing. The propagation of this technique has negatively affected CTA interpretation by rarely displaying the entire vessel in a single image/slab and by not providing the platform for crucial cross-sectional analysis. In addition there is a tendency to overestimate stenosis in the presence of (eccentric) calcified plaque and a potential for error because of the use of an incorrect slab thickness. If the slab thickness is less than the diameter of the coronary artery it may not show significant calcifications. On the other hand, if the slab is set too thick, it may highlight adjacent high-intensity voxels that do not belong to the current vessel of interest and may mask significant stenosis.

Advanced Viewing Tools

More detailed analysis of the CCTA dataset requires the semiautomatic extraction of the regions of interest.

Typically, the first step in any automated analysis or processing of cardiac CT images is the segmentation of the heart. During the segmentation process the individual voxels are assigned to a certain anatomy or to the background. Depending on its purpose, the segmentation step tries to identify several cardiac structures[17–21] or the whole anatomy of the heart.[22–29]

Segmentation algorithms can be divided into two classes: model-less and model-based approaches. The approaches of the former class typically consist of a chain of basic image processing operations, such as thresholding, region growing, edge detection, and so forth, and often require some form of user interaction (eg, placing seed points).[30,31] These methods can be time consuming and are prone to operator bias and inter-user variability. The algorithms in the model-based class extract the most descriptive statistical properties from a large pre-annotated training database or otherwise build an atlas based on this training set. The segmentation algorithm fits the model to a given dataset by varying the parameters of the model according to the predetermined statistical range. Most of these model-based approaches first perform a rough estimate of the location of the heart and then adapt a generalized model to the specific patient data by locally deforming the model. After the heart has been identified, the main anatomic structures, such as the atria, ventricles, myocardium, and large vessels, are segmented. In the last few years, these methods have matured in reliability and processing time, making them the method of choice for most digital workstations. (**Fig. 1**) shows an example of a fully automatic segmentation of a CTA volume in the most basic cardiac structures.

A disadvantage of these model-based approaches is that they may have difficulty dealing with anomalies or congenital deformities because the underlying model is not trained in these variations of the anatomy. In practice, this generally implies that the user is given the option to revert back to semi-intelligent manual (model-less) segmentation tools to handle these challenging cases. Regardless of the approach, the minimum segmentation should yield an effective extraction of the voxels that belong to the heart and its surrounding structures. Effectively, the spine, ribs, and other structures should have been removed. An example is given in **Fig. 2**, in which a lookup table is applied based on the Hounsfield values to make the visualization of the heart appear more realistic.

Extracting the Coronary Arteries from the CT Angiography Volume

The increased spatial and temporal resolution of MDCT has brought imaging and analysis of the coronary arteries within reach.[32–35] To enable automatic analysis of the coronary vessels, they need to be segmented from the CT data also.[36–40] The extraction of the coronary arteries from the cardiac CT data is generally started after the whole heart segmentation has been performed because it can provide clues to the location of the coronary arteries. The first step consists of extracting the tubular structures in the raw CT data. To facilitate this extraction process a separate representation is often generated in which the vessel-like structures are highlighted. An example of such a "vesselness"[41] filtered image is shown in **Fig. 3**.

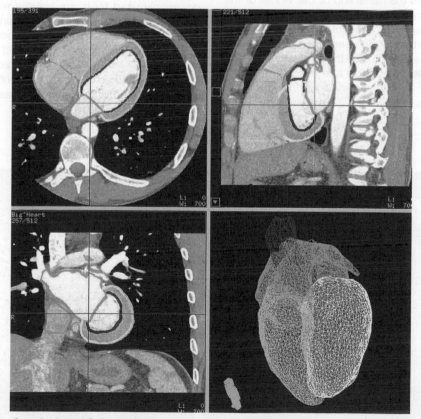

Fig. 1. Example of model-based fully automatic segmentation of the main cardiac structures from a CTA dataset. The extracted 3D surface mesh or model of the different structures is shown in the right lower frame; it is also superimposed on the three orthogonal slices in the cardiac CT volume.

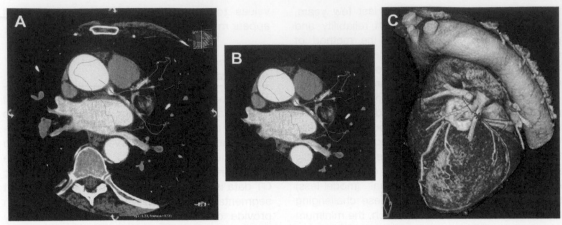

Fig. 2. Example of the segmented heart from a CTA volume. A slice from the original CTA scan (*A*), the same slice after segmenting the heart (*B*), and a color-coded volume rendering of the segmented heart (*C*).

The coronary artery tree is then traced in the vessel-enhanced data starting at the ostia, which could have been located during the preceding whole heart segmentation. The segmentation algorithm tries to follow the enhanced structures until it reaches the distal end of the vessel or the signal- or contrast-to-noise reaches a threshold. Most commercially available applications are capable of extracting the major coronary arteries, but let the operator provide the appropriate labels. Again, it is always possible to edit and extend the automatically found centerlines or to trace the entire vessels manually.

Multiplanar Reformats, Volume Rendering, and Quantitative Tools

Once the dataset is segmented and the coronary arteries extracted, there are a large number of tools available for visualization of the results. The most commonly used tools are volume rendering (VR, see also **Fig. 2**C) and the multiplanar reformats (MPRs). The VRs generally give an overview of the anatomic location of the arteries and their relation to other vessel structures. Highly calcified regions can also be marked to show the extent of the lesion. The often tortuous nature of the vessels does not

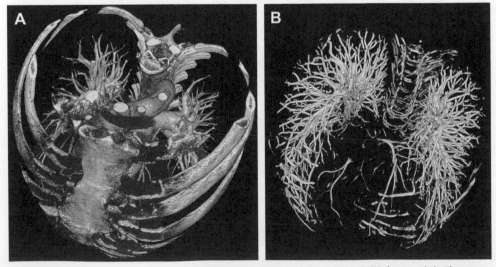

Fig. 3. Example of a vessel-enhanced image. A volume rendering of the original CT dataset (*A*). The same dataset after a vesselness filter was applied (*B*). The major coronary arteries are visible in the center of the volume.

allow them to be captured in their entirety in a single cut through the volume, however, even with a large slab size; this is the main reason for the existence of the family of MPRs. For example, curved MPRs enable the visualization of the entire course of the vessel, along with providing true distance measurements that are not subject to foreshortening. In addition, straightened MPRs enable the user to perform quantitative measurements, such as cross-sectional areas, stenosis, length of the vessel and the lesion, and so forth. **Fig. 4** gives an example of different types of MPRs and the derivation of some quantitative results.

The curved and straightened MPRs[42] of the entire coronary artery as shown in **Fig. 4** are the unequivocal format of choice and should be an absolute requirement. Total reliance on computer-generated MPRs is an invitation to error, however; center line review and correction by an experienced CT angiographer are essential. The operator must also be aware of the dependence of the diagnostic accuracy on the window center and width settings. Furthermore, the quantitative analysis of lesion characteristics is essential (**Fig. 4**C), and vastly preferable to the "eyeball" estimation routinely applied to CCA. Rotation of the MPRs around the extracted coronary artery center line allows the operator to display the smallest diameter and choose a normal reference area devoid of the positive remodeling that accompanies diseased segments and permits more meaningful calculations of percent diameter stenosis (**Fig. 4**A–C). The derived percent diameter stenosis should be rounded to the encompassing quartile (eg, 50%–75%) because the current spatial resolution of CCTA does not permit more precise quantitation. More importantly, the minimal luminal area (MLA) should be calculated from a cross-section derived from the straightened MPR (**Fig. 4**D, E) based on gradients from the contrast to the surrounding densities. MLA cannot be derived in sections with calcified plaque contiguous to the contrast. Hounsfield unit interrogation of different tissues may permit identification of negative-density lipid adjacent to the lumen that characterizes the thin cap fibroatheroma (**Fig. 4**F).

THE PREDICTIVE VALUE OF CORONARY CT ANGIOGRAPHY AND COMPARISON WITH CATHETER CORONARY ANGIOGRAPHY AND INTRAVASCULAR ULTRASOUND

Although there are a large number of segmentation and visualization tools available, it is not advisable to rely on a single representation and set of preset parameters. The accuracy of CCTA depends on

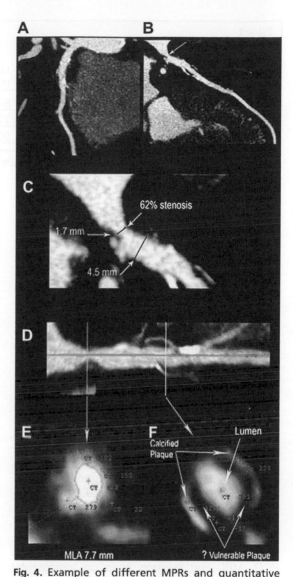

Fig. 4. Example of different MPRs and quantitative CCTA analysis. (*A*) Left anterior oblique and (*B*) right anterior oblique CTA MPR of the left anterior descending coronary artery. Significant stenosis apparent only in *B*. (*C*) Quantitative measurement of the stenotic area in *B*. (*D*) Straightened MPR with cursors drawn through the proximal stenosis and the more distal complex plaque. (*E*) Cross-sectional analysis of the proximal stenosis. The numbers represent the HU of the pixels marked by the adjacent plus signs. The contour is drawn around the lumen on the basis of the gradation of HU. The luminal area within the contour is 7.7 mm², which is more than adequate to allow proper blood flow. (*F*) Multiple tissue densities are demonstrated, including low and negative-density nonobstructive plaque, with negative HU, suggesting a potentially vulnerable thin cap fibroatheroma.

Table 1
Diagnostic performance of 64-slice CT angiography

Level of Analysis	Prevalence of Disease (%)	Sensitivity (%)	Specificity (%)	Positive Predictive Value (%)	Negative Predictive Value (%)
Patient-based	68	99	64	86	97
Vessel-based	26	95	77	59	98
Segment-based	9	88	90	47	99

From Cox CE. CTA reliably rules out CAD, specificity still an issue. Available at http://www.tctmd.com/Show.aspx?id=75478. Accessed April 3, 2009; with permission.

a highly variable learning curve for achieving adequate processing and interpretative skills. In recent years, single- and multicenter studies have investigated the use of CCTA to predict the absence or occurrence of significant CAD in symptomatic patients who had intermediate risk for disease. Overall, these studies have consistently shown a high negative predictive value (>95%),[1,2,4–6] whereas the positive predictive values are more variable and depend on the disease prevalence.[43,44] A recent prospective multicenter multivendor study on the use of 64-slice CTA in patients who had stable or unstable angina[7] made a distinction between patient-based, vessel-based, and segment-based performance and showed impressive results for the negative predictive value in all analyses (**Table 1**), with declining positive predictive values as the disease prevalence decreased.

The major concern with most of these comparative studies is the choice of the gold standard. Traditionally, all the noninvasive diagnostic technologies, including nuclear cardiology, stress ECG, MRI, and positron emission tomography perfusion imaging, have used a cutoff of greater than 50% diameter stenosis on CCA as the gold standard, despite the limitations inherent in 2D lumenology, clearly demonstrated by intravascular ultrasound (IVUS). The most important limitations are: inability to define normal reference areas, limited number of acquisitions, and reliance on percentage diameter stenosis rather than MLA. Nonetheless, CCA has also been used as the gold standard for CCTA, even though CCTA has more in common with IVUS, such as the availability of cross-sectional wall and lumen (see[45] and **Table 2** for details). In particular, the ability to calculate minimal luminal area,[46,47] to view a stenosis from an infinite number of angles, and to characterize plaque[48–50] are IVUS characteristics that greatly affect PCI. Despite the limited spatial and temporal resolution of CCTA, the noninvasive and less-expensive acquisitions and the radiation dose reduction offered by prospective imaging are distinct advantages. Although not a coronary imaging tool, myocardial perfusion imaging is associated with more radiation (11–23 mSv)[51] and is still recommended before CCTA in the diagnostic

Table 2
Comparison of catheter coronary angiography, intravascular ultrasound, and coronary CT angiography

	CCA	IVUS	CCTA
Spatial resolution	200 µm	100–150 µm	350 µm
Temporal resolution	5–10 ms	NA	40–100 ms
Imaging	Projection/2DLumen	Cross-sectionalWall and lumen	Cross-sectionalWall and lumen
Parameter	% Diameter stenosis	Minimum luminal area	Minimum luminal area
Plaque character	Not applicable	Readily available	Readily available
Imaging area	All segments	Limited segments	All segments
Acquisition	Invasive	Highly invasive	Noninvasive
Radiation	5 mSv	>5 mSv (part of PCI)	2–20 mSv
Cost	High	High	Low

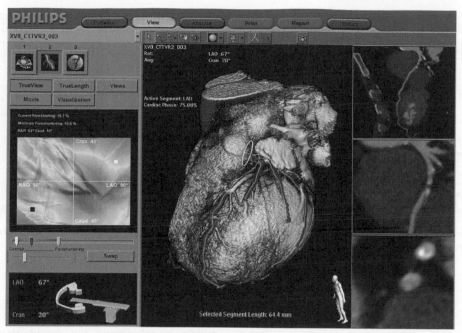

Fig. 5. In-room presentation of CTA data using VR and MPR visualization techniques.

paradigm despite its inferior sensitivity and specificity for detecting significant obstructive disease.[52]

PERIOPERATIVE USE OF CORONARY CT ANGIOGRAPHY

If the findings on the CCTA result in the decision to proceed with the cardiac catheterization, then the challenge becomes transferring the information gathered thus far to aid in the decision-making process. This section discusses some options and requirements of the in-room use of the CCTA data beginning with basic use and concluding with future applications.

Adapting the Diagnostic Catheterization

In general, a complete diagnostic catheterization is performed regardless of the CCTA findings, if only to confirm these and obtain information that is not readily present in the CT scan, such as the assessment of blood flow and the presence of collaterals. The CT data may suggest a series of C-arm angles that may be different than the routine views commonly used by the cardiologist. Depending on the familiarity of the physician with the CT data and the quality of the scan, an even larger deviation from the routine standard views may be used. At the extreme end, the entire diagnostic catheterization may be completely guided by the CT. In this patient-specific application, the CT dictates the viewing angles or (dual-axis) rotational acquisitions that would optimally yield the vessel segments of interest. Apart from confirming the diagnosis based on CT, it offers potential working views to perform the actual intervention. In addition, the amount of time, contrast, and radiation needed to complete the diagnostic scan may be reduced. In the future, the cardiologist may even refrain from injecting the right coronary

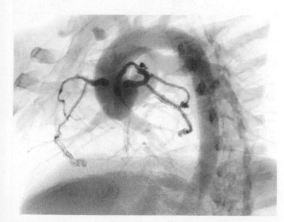

Fig. 6. Example of a digitally reconstructed radiograph (DRR) based on a segmented CCTA dataset.

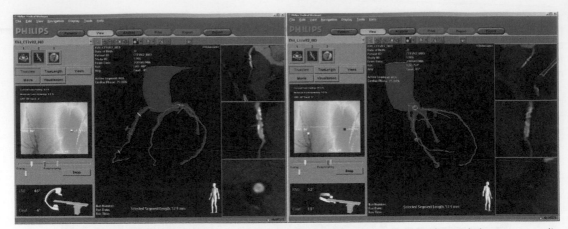

Fig. 7. Example of visualizing the CT-based coronary tree from different viewing angles and the corresponding C-arm gantry configuration.

altogether if the CCTA only shows disease in the left coronary system.

In-room Visualization and Manipulation

In the anticipation that CCTA will play a more dominant role in the future, several companies have products available or are planning functionality that facilitates the transfer and the use of the CT data and some of their quantitative information in the cardiac catheterization laboratory (eg, Shina Systems, Siemens Healthcare, GE Healthcare, and Philips Healthcare). Especially for complex vasculature, chronic total occlusions (CTO), unusual anatomy, and strange take-off angles, it has been shown to be beneficial to have the CT data available in the room.[53–56] Because the ability for in-room manipulation of the CT data and their derived information by the interventionalist during the diagnostic and PCI portion is limited, it is key to show the essentials of the CT information during the critical portions of the procedure. An example is given in **Fig. 5**.

In **Fig. 5** a combination of VR and MPRs is shown, specific for the lesion of interest. If a segmentation of the CT into different tissue types (eg, blood, muscle, bone) or anatomic segments is performed (eg, spine, ribs, cardiac chambers), this information can be used to better reveal the areas of interest. From the table side the operator has the opportunity to select the coronary artery of interest and define the vessel segment of interest. In the lower left panel the C-arm configuration is shown that corresponds with the current viewing angle of the CT dataset. The color-coded rectangle on the left

middle panel shows the foreshortening map combined with an overlap map (see the article by Garcia and Movassaghi elsewhere in this issue), which can offer other properties to aid in finding the optimal working view for the actual intervention.

Furthermore, a particular X-ray projection view can be simulated based on the segmented CT data using digitally reconstructed radiographs (DRR). Advances in graphical processing unit programming and computing power allow for extremely fast rendering times of these DRRs.[57] **Fig. 6** gives an example of such a simulated

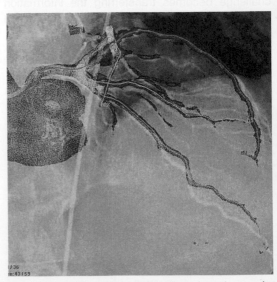

Fig. 8. Example of a registration based on the coronary arteries.

view, where the bony structures and the coronary tree as derived from the CT are purposefully shown. An advantage of this type of rendering technique is that it displays the data in a fashion more familiar to the interventionalist.

Recently, some researchers and manufacturers have moved toward an even more intimate integration between the X-ray acquisition equipment and the preoperative 3D dataset. As the first step, the C-arm angulations of the X-ray gantry are transmitted to the 3D workstation to allow the CT data to be viewed in the current gantry orientation. With such a capability, the clinician has the opportunity to move the C-arm to a desired position while the 3D CT data (now coupled with the X-ray acquisition equipment) are rotated and rendered accordingly.

Fig. 7 shows an example of the CT-rendered coronary tree from several different viewing angles and their corresponding gantry configuration (see also Video 1, available in the online version of this article at: http://www.cardiology.theclinics.com). As an alternative, some systems allow a physician to select any viewing angle solely based on the CT data–derived optimal view map without considering the gantry's mechanical limitation, environmental setup, and patient's condition. As a result, the computer-predicted viewing angle might not be achievable because of the patient size, obstruction by other equipment

or the table-bed, steepness of the viewing angle, and other complicating factors.

Taking this one step further, the status of gantry configuration, including the table position, height, detector size, source to detector distance (SDD), and so forth, are recorded and instantaneously sent to the control unit. In these applications the configuration of the gantry is tracked in real time to yield projection images of the 3D coronary vasculature to simulate conventional angiographic views without administration of additional contrast and x-ray dose to facilitate the percutaneous coronary intervention.

Image Fusion

Future significant advances will require actual fusion of the CCTA and CCA images, thereby eliminating the persistent problem of exactly translating a CCTA-directed intervention to the CCA-defined coronary artery. CCTA has the potential to be used for roadmapping, by which the stream of live X-ray images are superimposed on the volume-rendered representation of the (segmented) CCTA data. Although the presumed benefits of these roadmapping applications are currently under investigation, they will likely prove to be crucial for more accurate stent placement and in the treatment of CTOs.

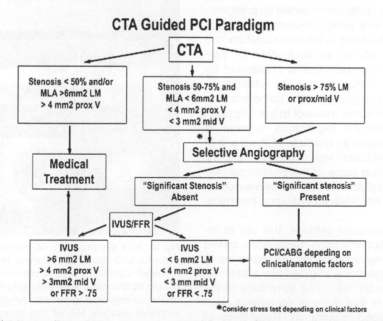

Fig. 9. CTA-guided PCI paradigm. CABG, coronary artery bypass grafting; FFR, fractional flow reserve; LM, left main; V, vessel.

Registration

To perform image fusion, it is essential to establish a mapping between the CCTA dataset and the X-ray gantry. In this registration process the anatomic features that are apparent in both modalities are used to compensate for the differences in patient orientation. Typically a registration algorithm consists of a similarity measure, indicating the quality of a given spatial mapping, and an optimization algorithm, which iteratively searches the optimum of the similarity measure. Currently most of these roadmapping applications use either bony landmarks, such as the ribs and spine, the pulmonary veins, or the contrast-filled coronary arteries, whereas other approaches make use of the DRRs again to measure the match between the fluoroscopy images and the CT data.[58] Because most MDCTs are equipped with a concave table, however, registration using a simple or rigid rotation and translation would result in a suboptimal solution. Instead, a more computationally expensive non-affine registration method is used. The resultant hybrid CT–radiographic image has several clinical applications, such as radiotherapy planning and verification, surgery planning and guidance, and minimally invasive vascular treatment in peripheral and neurovascular interventions. In the cardiac domain, most work with respect to roadmapping applications has focused on electrophysiological interventions,[59,60] and only recently some clinical applications related to the treatment of coronary artery disease are being explored.[54,61–63] Although the roadmapping applications based on preoperative CT and MR have yielded impressive accuracy and several applications in neurovasculature and peripheral interventions, its application for performing coronary interventions is challenged by cardiac and respiratory motion. In addition, to salvage the earlier registration the catheterization laboratory table requires a sensor to track its position or an automatic registration process is needed. **Fig. 8** shows an example of the result of an automatic registration technique on a patient's dataset, highlighting some of the challenges (see also Video 2, available in the online version of this article at: http://www.cardiology.theclinics.com).

In some experimental settings, the use of in-room CT-like reconstruction techniques based on rotational X-ray acquisitions (as explained in the chapter on rotational angiography elsewhere in this issue) can be used. The advantage of the latter approach is that there is no explicit need for an image-based registration. Regardless of these issues, image fusion shows great promise, particularly in complex interventions in which the CT data add complementary information to the radiographic images.

CURRENT AND FUTURE APPLICATIONS OF CORONARY CT ANGIOGRAPHY TO PERCUTANEOUS CORONARY INTERVENTION

In the previous section, the technology and tools that are currently available (or under development) to the interventionalist were discussed. This section gives some practical examples of how some of these tools can be applied and how they

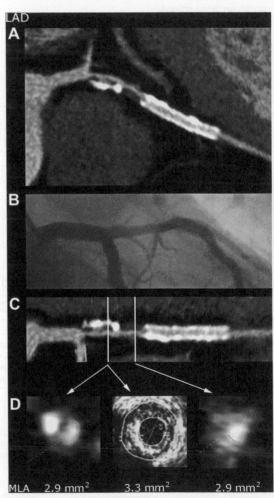

Fig. 10. In a symptomatic 64-year-old man who had previous LAD stent, CCTA curved MPR of the LAD (*A*) revealed significant diffuse narrowing from the LAD ostium to the stent, with only mild narrowing evident on the corresponding catheter angiography (*B*). Cross-sectional analysis (*D*) of the straightened MPR (*C*) demonstrated significantly reduced MLA of 2.9 mm², confirmed by IVUS (*D*), and followed by PCI.

have the potential to affect the treatment plan and the execution of the PCI after a positive CT is found.

Percutaneous Coronary Intervention Patient Selection and Identification of Significant Lesions

The paradigm shown in **Fig. 9** replaces stress testing with CTA as the first test in the evaluation of a patient who has CAD, and relies more on the IVUS MLA criteria than percent diameter stenosis.[55] Discrepancies between CCTA and CCA stenosis characterization are adjudicated by either IVUS or fractional flow reserve.[64] In

Fig. 10, diffuse narrowing of the entire proximal left anterior descending (LAD) was evident on CCTA, with an MLA of 2.9 mm². CCA revealed only minimal narrowing, highlighting its difficulty in identifying diffusely narrowed segments that, by definition, have no normal reference areas. IVUS clearly corroborated the CCTA findings.[55]

The same principle applies to in-stent restenosis (ISR). In **Fig. 10**, uniform in-stent contrast density indicates absence of significant neointimal hyperplasia. Severe in-stent hypodensity is noted in **Fig. 11**, consistent with significant narrowing, not apparent on CCA but confirmed by IVUS.[55]

Procedure Planning: Stent Sizing

CCTA facilitates precise determination of the area to be covered based on measurement of the length

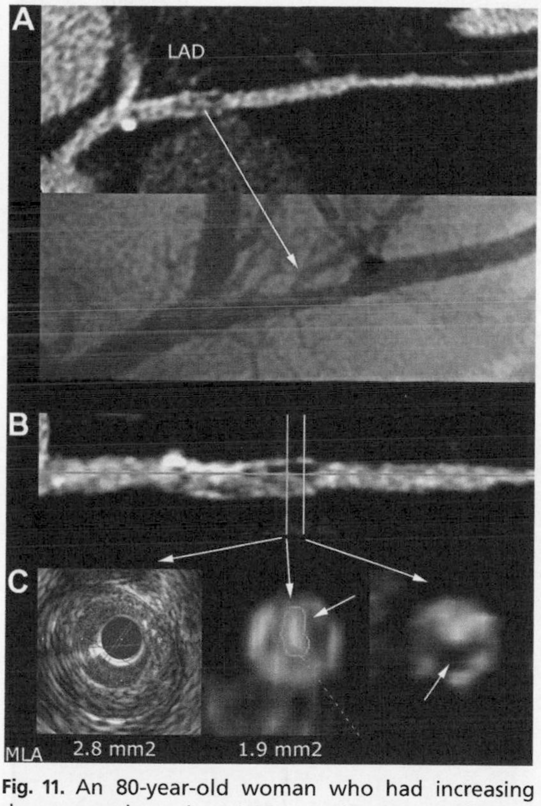

Fig. 11. An 80-year-old woman who had increasing dyspnea and previous LAD stenting was evaluated. CTA revealed severe hypodensity consistent with significant ISR (*A, top*) that appeared to be only moderately severe on catheter angiography (*A, bottom*). Cross-sectional analysis (*C*) of the straightened MPR (*B*) in two adjacent areas of the stent demonstrated the hypodensity characteristic of neointimal hyperplasia (*arrows*) and severely decreased MLA, confirmed by IVUS (*C*). PCI was performed. In-stent MLA calculation is rarely possible. Blooming artifact from the dense stent material almost always precludes accurate measurement; ISR is diagnosed by qualitative density levels.

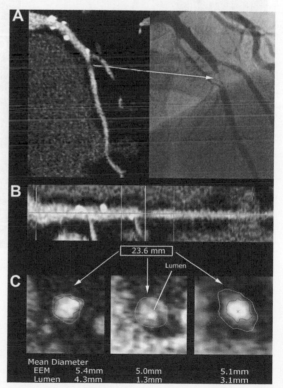

Fig. 12. In a 66-year-old man who had increasing angina, subtotal LAD occlusion (*arrow*) was noted on the CTA (*A, left*) and on the coronary angiography (*A, right*). Proximal and distal stent landing zones, 23.6 mm apart, were chosen on the straightened MPR (*B*). Mean luminal diameters for the landing zones were determined by cross-sectional analysis to be 4.4 and 3.1 mm, respectively (*C*). PCI was performed using a 25 × 3.5 mm stent, with post inflation of the proximal segment to 4.5 mm to achieve full apposition.

of diseased vessel wall that warrants exclusion rather than on an estimation of the lumen stenosis length on CCA. Proximal and distal landing zones can be axially sized and post dilation planned, as in **Fig. 12**. The angle of least foreshortening of the stenosis can be selected based on the CT. Presumed vulnerable low-density plaques on the stenosis margins may be covered also, even though there are no supporting data.

Procedure Planning: Chronic Total Occlusions

CCTA has shown to be extremely beneficial for the PCI of CTOs,[53] and has been invaluable in

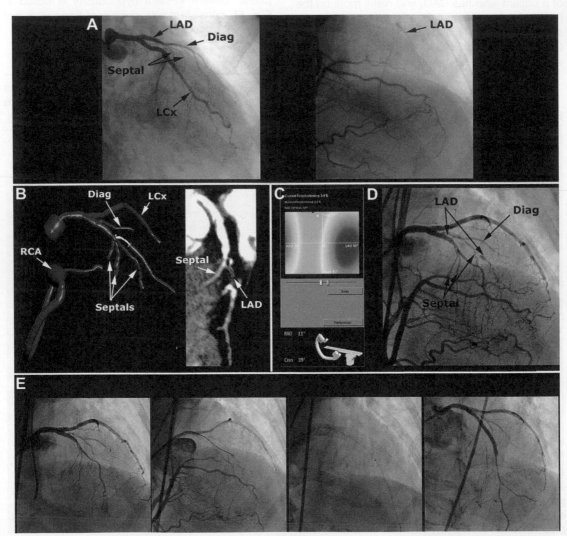

Fig. 13. Selective angiography demonstrated flush occlusion of the LAD with partial collateral filling from the right coronary artery (*A*) in a symptomatic 65-year-old woman who had anterior ischemia. After 6 months of persistent symptoms, CTA-guided intervention was planned. Curved MPR readily visualized the occluded LAD segment (*B*). CTA mapping (CT TrueView, Philips Healthcare) of the left coronary artery and all its branches (*C*) was imported to the catheterization laboratory monitor and electronically linked to the C-arm. The C-arm was rotated, with accompanying automatic rotation of the TrueView map to the angle predetermined by the CCTA to best demonstrate the origin and course of the chronic total occlusion without overlapping branches. Simultaneous injection of the right and left coronary arteries (*D*) was performed. With TrueView guidance, the guidewire was introduced to the precise origin of the flush occlusion, followed by successful recanalization and further stenting of the distal vessel 6 weeks later (*E*). Diag, diagonal; LAD, left anterior descending; LCx, left circumflex; RCA = right coronary artery.

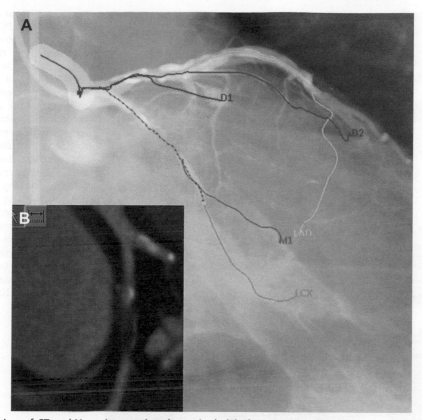

Fig. 14. (*A*) Fusion of CT and X-ray images (roadmapping). (*B*) The corresponding MPR.

identifying the often angiographically invisible occluded segment, which can always be tracked by CCTA. Of equal importance is preprocedural determination of the best angle to approach the CTO, using branch vessels as landmarks, as demonstrated in **Fig. 13**.

A typical example of CTO revascularization using image fusion is demonstrated in **Fig. 14** (see also Video 3, available in the online version of this article at: http://www.cardiology.theclinics.com). The CCA reveals the vessel cutoff, whereas the superimposed CT images from a similar viewing angle demonstrate the occluded segment and the remainder of the left circumflex artery, which is filled by collaterals. Successful restoration of flow was accomplished by the antegrade technique. Ultimately, the cardiac phase of the CT image would be matched to the cardiac phase of the radiographic data. Currently the CT images are shown in a preselected static cardiac phase; the coronary arteries in the X-ray image display a periodic motion around the coronary arteries, which were segmented from the CT data.

Plaque Evaluation and Identification of High-risk Lesions

Ulcerated and ruptured plaques (**Fig. 15**) and presumed thin-cap fibroatheromas can be identified by CCTA (see **Fig. 4**). If ongoing studies prospectively localize ischemic events to vulnerable areas and are accompanied by data supporting stenting these areas, CCTA may be used to noninvasively localize the high-risk lesion before intervention.

SUMMARY

That CCTA will significantly alter the practice of PCI is abundantly clear; it is still in its relative infancy, with forthcoming technological advances likely to accelerate the pace of change. The prerequisite human ingredient is a change in mind-set, an acknowledgment that the traditional reliance on CCA is limiting, despite the decades of data accumulated in the catheterization laboratory. Had IVUS been available from the beginning of angiography, there is little doubt that it would

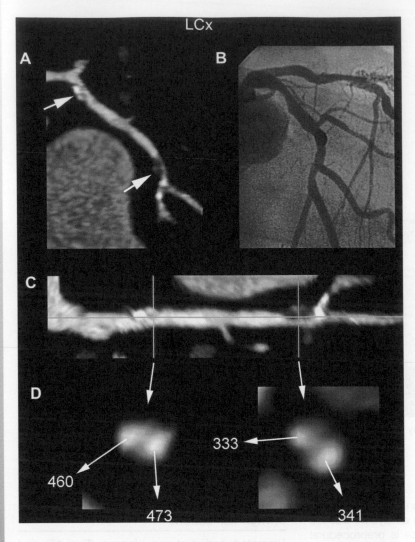

Fig. 15. A 52-year-old man who had previous PCI underwent CCTA (*A*) after presenting with recurrent chest pain. In the proximal left circumflex (LCx) (*arrow*), a complex plaque was noted, containing calcified plaque and a second component extrinsic to the lumen, with density similar to contrast. In the mid LCx, a similar extraluminal density was noted (*arrow*). CCA performed 2 weeks later (*B*) did not reveal these findings and the mid LCx stenosis was not apparent. Cross-sectional analysis (*D*) of the straightened MPR (*C*) confirmed the extraluminal densities to be similar to contrast, consistent with plaque rupture at both sites.

have been the gold standard. CCTA provides the opportunity to incorporate the unique insights offered by IVUS into a universally available noninvasive tool that can now be brought directly into the catheterization laboratory. The likely outcome is transformation of the catheterization laboratory into a streamlined interventional suite, using fused CCTA and CCA data in an interactive format.

APPENDIX: SUPPLEMENTARY MATERIAL

Supplementary material can be found in the online version, at: doi:10.1016/j.ccl.2009.04.002.

REFERENCES

1. Hoffmann MH, Shi H, Schmitz BL, et al. Noninvasive coronary angiography with multislice computed tomography. JAMA 2005;293(20):2471–8 [erratum in: JAMA. 2005 Sep 14;294(10):1208].

2. Raff GL, Gallagher MJ, O'Neill WW, et al. Diagnostic accuracy of noninvasive coronary angiography using 64-slice spiral computed tomography. J Am Coll Cardiol 2005;46(3):552–7.

3. Leschka S, Alkadhi H, Plass A, et al. Accuracy of MSCT coronary angiography with 64 slice technology: first experience. Eur Heart J 2005;26: 1482–7.

4. Garcia MJ, Lessick J, Hoffmann MH. Accuracy of 16-row multidetector computed tomography for the assessment of coronary artery stenosis. JAMA 2006;296(4):403–11.

5. Watkins MW, Hesse B, Green CE, et al. Detection of coronary artery stenosis using 40-channel computed tomography with multi-segment reconstruction. Am J Cardiol 2007;99(2):175–81 [Epub 2006 Nov 14].

6. Budoff MJ, Dowe D, Jollis JG, et al. Diagnostic performance of 64-multidetector row coronary computed tomographic angiography for evaluation

of coronary artery stenosis in individuals without known coronary artery disease: results from the prospective multicenter ACCURACY (Assessment by Coronary Computed Tomographic Angiography of Individuals Undergoing Invasive Coronary Angiography) trial. J Am Coll Cardiol 2008;52(21): 1724–32.

7. Meijboom WB, Meijs MFL, Schuijf JD. Diagnostic accuracy of 64-slice computed tomography coronary angiography: a prospective, multicenter, multivendor study. J Am Coll Cardiol 2008;52:2135–44.

8. Hendel RC, Patel MR, Kramer CM, et al. ACCF/ACR/ SCCT/SCMR/ASNC/NASCI/SCAI/SIR 2006 appropriateness criteria for cardiac computed tomography and cardiac magnetic resonance imaging: a report of the American College of Cardiology Foundation Quality Strategic Directions Committee Appropriateness Criteria Working Group, American College of Radiology, Society of Cardiovascular Computed Tomography, Society for Cardiovascular Magnetic Resonance, American Society of Nuclear Cardiology, North American Society for Cardiac Imaging, Society for Cardiovascular Angiography and Interventions, and Society of Interventional Radiology. J Am Coll Cardiol 2006;48(7):1475–97. 1.

9. Maruyama T, Motoyama S, Anno H, et al. Noninvasive coronary angiography with a prototype 256-row area detector computed tomography system: comparison with conventional invasive coronary angiography. J Am Coll Cardiol 2008;51:773–5.

10. Husmann L, Valenta I, Gaemperli O, et al. Feasibility of low-dose coronary CT angiography: first experience with prospective ECG-gating. Eur Heart J 2007;29(2):191–7.

11. Earls JP, Berman EL, Urban BA, et al. Prospectively gated transverse coronary CT angiography versus retrospectively gated helical technique: improved image quality and reduced radiation dose. Radiology 2008;246(3):742–53.

12. Shuman WP, Branch KR, May JM, et al. Prospective versus retrospective ECG gating for 64-detector CT of the coronary arteries: comparison of image quality and patient radiation dose. Radiology 2008; 248(2):431–7.

13. Hirai N, Horiguchi J, Fujioka C, et al. Prospective versus retrospective ECG-gated 64-detector coronary CT angiography: assessment of image quality, stenosis, and radiation dose. Radiology 2008; 248(2):424–30.

14. Klass O, Jeltsch M, Feuerlein S, et al. Prospectively-gated axial CT coronary angiography: preliminary experiences with a novel low-dose technique. Eur Radiol 2009;19(4):829–36.

15. Scheffel H, Alkadhi H, Leschka S, et al. Low-dose CT coronary angiography in the step-and-shoot mode: diagnostic performance. Heart 2008;94: 1132–7.

16. Maruyama T, Takada M, Hasuike T, et al. Radiation dose reduction and coronary assessability of prospective electrocardiogram-gated computed tomography coronary angiography. Comparison with retrospective electrocardiogram-gated helical scan. J Am Coll Cardiol 2008;52:1450–5.

17. Okuyama T, Ehara S, Shirai N, et al. Usefulness of three-dimensional automated quantification of left ventricular mass, volume, and function by 64-slice computed tomography. J Cardiol 2008;52(3): 276–84.

18. Spoeck A, Bonatti J, Friedrich GJ, et al. Evaluation of left ventricular function by 64-multidetector computed tomography in patients undergoing totally endoscopic coronary artery bypass grafting. Heart Surg Forum 2008;11(4):E218–24.

19. Cristoforetti A, Faes L, Ravelli F, et al. Isolation of the left atrial surface from cardiac multi-detector CT images based on marker controlled watershed segmentation. Med Eng Phys 2008;30(1):48–58 [Epub 2007 Mar 27].

20. Sun W, Qetin M, Chan R, et al. Segmenting and tracking the left ventricle by learning the dynamics in cardiac images. Inf Process Med Imaging 2005; 19:553–65.

21. Lynch M, Ghita O, Whelan PF. Left-ventricle myocardium segmentation using a coupled level-set with a priori knowledge. Comput Med Imaging Graph 2006;30(4):255–62.

22. Zheng Y, Barbu A, Georgescu B, et al. Four-chamber heart modeling and automatic segmentation for 3-D cardiac CT volumes using marginal space learning and steerable features. IEEE Trans Med Imaging 2008;27(11):1668–81.

23. Ecabert O, Peters J, Schramm H, et al. Automatic model-based segmentation of the heart in CT images. IEEE Trans Med Imaging 2008;27(9): 1189–201.

24. Wijesooriya K, Weiss E, Dill V, et al. Quantifying the accuracy of automated structure segmentation in 4D CT images using a deformable image registration algorithm. Med Phys 2008;35(4):1251–60.

25. Fleureau J, Garreau M, Boulmier D, et al. 3D multi-object segmentation of cardiac MSCT imaging by using a multi-agent approach. Conf Proc IEEE Eng Med Biol Soc 2007;2007:6004–7.

26. Renno MS, Shang Y, Sweeney J, et al. Segmentation of 4D cardiac images: investigation on statistical shape models. Conf Proc IEEE Eng Med Biol Soc 2006;1:3086–9.

27. Lorenz C, von Berg J. A comprehensive shape model of the heart. Med Image Anal 2006;10(4): 657–70 [Epub 2006 May 18].

28. van Assen HC, Danilouchkine MG, Dirksen MS, et al. A 3-D active shape model driven by fuzzy inference: application to cardiac CT and MR. IEEE Trans Inf Technol Biomed 2008;12(5):595–605.

29. Cho J, Benkeser PJ. Cardiac segmentation by a velocity-aided active contour model. Comput Med Imaging Graph 2006;30(1):31–41 [Epub 2005 Dec 27].

30. Higgins WE, Chung N, Ritman EL. Extraction of left-ventricular chamber from 3-D CT images of the heart. IEEE Trans Med Imaging 1990;9(4):384–94.

31. Redwood AB, Camp JJ, Robb RA. Semiautomatic segmentation of the heart from CT images based on intensity and morphological features. Conference Proceedings of the SPIE 2005;5747:1713–9.

32. Marquering HA, Dijkstra J, de Koning PJ, et al. Towards quantitative analysis of coronary CTA. Int J Cardiovasc Imaging 2005;21(1):73–84.

33. Saur SC, Alkadhi H, Desbiolles L, et al. Automatic detection of calcified coronary plaques in computed tomography data sets. Med Image Comput Comput Assist Interv Int Conf Med Image Comput Comput Assist Interv 2008;11(Pt 1):170–7.

34. Isgum I, Rutten A, Prokop M, et al. Detection of coronary calcifications from computed tomography scans for automated risk assessment of coronary artery disease. Med Phys 2007;34(4):1450–61.

35. Horiguchi J, Fujioka C, Kiguchi M, et al. Soft and intermediate plaques in coronary arteries: how accurately can we measure CT attenuation using 64-MDCT? AJR Am J Roentgenol 2007;189(4): 981–8.

36. Bousse A, Boldak C, Toumoulin C, et al. Coronary extraction and characterization in multi-detector computed tomography. ITBM-RBM 2006;27(5–6): 217–26.

37. Fallavollita P, Cheriet F. Towards an automatic coronary artery segmentation algorithm. Conf Proc IEEE Eng Med Biol Soc 2006;3037–40.

38. Fallavollita P, Cheriet F. Optimal 3D reconstruction of coronary arteries for 3D clinical assessment. Comput Med Imaging Graph 2008;32(6):476–87.

39. Mueller D, Maeder A. Robust semi-automated path extraction for visualising stenosis of the coronary arteries. Comput Med Imaging Graph 2008;32(6): 463–75.

40. Zambal S, Hladuvka J, Kanitsar A, et al. and for automatic coronary artery tracking. Presented at: MICCAI 2008 Workshop. New York: September, 2008.

41. Frangi AF, Niessen WJ, Vincken KL, et al. Multiscale vessel enhancement filtering. Conference Proceedings of the first MICCAI. Cambridge, MA: 1998;130–7.

42. Kanitsar A, Fleischmann D, Wegenkittl R, et al. - CPR curved planar reformation. VIS '02: IEEE Proc. Conf. Visualization '02, Boston, Ma, USA.

43. Hamon M, Biondi-Zoccai GGL, Malagutti P, et al. Diagnostic performance of multislice spiral computed tomography of coronary arteries as compared with conventional invasive coronary angiography. A meta-analysis. J Am Coll Cardiol 2006;48:1896–910.

44. Hamon M, Morello R, Riddell JW, et al. Diagnostic performance of 16- versus 64-section spiral CT compared with invasive coronary angiography—meta-analysis. Radiology 2007;245(3):720–31.

45. Cox CE. CTA reliably rules out CAD, specificity still an issue. Available at: http://www.tctmd.com/Show. aspx?id=75478. Accessed April 3, 2009.

46. Caussin C, Larchez C, Ghostine S, et al. Comparison of coronary minimal lumen area quantification by sixty-four-slice computed tomography versus intravascular ultrasound for intermediate stenosis. Am J Cardiol 2006;98:871–6.

47. Okabe T, Weigold WG, Mintz GS, et al. Comparison of intravascular ultrasound to contrast-enhanced 64-slice computed tomography to assess the significance of angiographically ambiguous coronary narrowings. Am J Cardiol 2008;102:994–1001.

48. Pundziute G, Schuijf JD, Jukema JW, et al. Evaluation of plaque characteristics in acute coronary syndromes: non-invasive assessment with multislice computed tomography and invasive evaluation with intravascular ultrasound radiofrequency data analysis. Eur Heart J 2008;29(19):2373–81.

49. Springer I, Dewey M. Comparison of multislice computed tomography with intravascular ultrasound for detection and characterization of coronary artery plaques: a systematic review. Eur J Radiol 2008;. [epub ahead of print].

50. Pundziute G, Schuijf JD, Jukema JW, et al. Head-to-head comparison of coronary plaque evaluation between multislice computed tomography and intravascular ultrasound radiofrequency data analysis. J Am Coll Cardiol Intv 2008;1:176–82.

51. Thompson RC, Cullom SJ. Issues regarding radiation dosage of cardiac nuclear and radiography procedures. J Nucl Cardiol 2006;13:19–23.

52. Fleischmann KE, Hunink MG, Kuntz KM, et al. Exercise echocardiography or exercise SPECT imaging? A meta-analysis of diagnostic test performance. JAMA 1998;280:913–20.

53. Mollet NR, Hoye A, Lemos PA, et al. Value of preprocedure multislice computed tomographic coronary angiography to predict the outcome of percutaneous recanalization of chronic total occlusions. Am J Cardiol 2005;95:240–3.

54. Garcia JA, Eng MH, Wink O, et al. Clinical review: image guidance of percutaneous coronary and structural heart disease interventions using a computed tomography and fluoroscopy integration. Vascular Disease Management 2007;4(3):89–97.

55. Hecht HS. Applications of multislice coronary computed tomography angiography to percutaneous coronary intervention: how did we ever do without it? Catheter Cardiovasc Interv 2008;71: 490–503.

56. Otsuka M, Sugahara S, Umeda K, et al. Utility of mul-tislice computed tomography as a strategic tool for complex percutaneous coronary interventions. Int J Cadiovasc Imaging 2008;24:201–10.

57. Russakoff DB, Rohlfing T, Mori K, et al. Fast genera-tion of digitally reconstructed radiographs using attenuation fields with application to 2D-3D image registration. IEEE Trans Med Imaging 2005;24(11): 1441–54.

58. Weese J, Buzug TM, Lorenz C, et al. An approach to 2D/3D registration of a vertebra in 2D X-ray fluoros-copies with 3D CT images. Springer: CVRMed 1997; 119–12.

59. Sra J, Narayan G, Krum D, et al. Computed tomo-graphy-fluoroscopy image integration-guided catheter ablation of atrial fibrillation. J Cardiovasc Electrophysiol 2007;18(4):409–14.

60. Knecht S, Skali H, O'Neill MD, et al. Computed tomography-fluoroscopy overlay evaluation during catheter ablation of left atrial arrhythmia. Europace 2008;10(8):931–8.

61. Turgeon GA, Lehmann G, Guiraudon G, et al. 2D-3D registration of coronary angiograms for cardiac plan-ning and guidance. Med Phys 2005;32(12):3737–49.

62. Hecht HS, Roubin G. Usefulness of computed tomography guided percutaneous coronary inter-vention. Am J Cardiol 2007;99:871–5.

63. Garcia JA, Bhakta S, Kay J, et al. On-line multi-slice computed tomography interactive overlay with conventional X-ray: a new and advanced imaging fusion concept. Int J Cardiol 2009;133(3):e101–5.

64. Tobis J, Azarbal B, Slavin L. Assessment of interme-diate severity coronary lesions in the catheterization laboratory. J Am Coll Cardiol 2007;49:839–48.

Intravascular Ultrasound Registration/ Integration with Coronary Angiography

Nico Bruining, PhD*, Sebastiaan de Winter, BSc,
Patrick W. Serruys, MD, PhD

KEYWORDS
- Angiography • Intravascular ultrasound • Coronary
- Interventions • Image processing

Coronary angiography has undergone tremendous development since the first catheterization by Forssmann in 1929 and the first selective coronary angiography by Sones in 1960.[1] Despite recent strong interest in other coronary imaging modalities such as multislice computed tomography (MSCT), coronary angiography is still the workhorse for the diagnosis of coronary artery disease and for guiding interventional therapies (**Fig. 1**). The two-dimensional (2D) representation of the coronary lumen as a silhouette has well-recognized limitations, however.[2–4]

Since its introduction[5] in the late 1980s and early 1990s, intravascular ultrasound (IVUS) has proved a valuable additional coronary imaging tool used in conjunction with angiography.[2–4,6] It provides the clinician with highly detailed cross-sectional images of the coronary vessel wall morphology[7] that cannot be visualized by angiography alone. Many studies showed that the use of IVUS as a guidance tool for interventions can improve clinical outcome.[8,9] Furthermore, IVUS is the reference method used in many clinical trials studying coronary artery disease[10] and evaluating new coronary therapies, both pharmaceutical[11,12] (eg, progression/regression studies)[13] and interventional.[14] Although new additional imaging methods such as optical coherence tomography[15] and minimally invasive coronary MSCT[16,17] are gaining attention and are used increasingly, they are still in the exploratory phase. IVUS, however, is a

well-established, validated, mature, and safe technology.[18]

Because angiography, also called "luminography," visualizes the coronary artery lumen as a projected 2D silhouette, in contrast to IVUS, which displays a small cross-sectional view of the coronary vessel perpendicular to its catheter path (see **Fig. 1**), a visualization combining both modalities would be ideal. Unfortunately, although IVUS has been around for almost 20 years, until recently the technological infrastructure within the catheterization laboratory did not allow the easy clinical use of such combined visualization. In the era of angiography using film and IVUS recorded on videotape, combined visualization was possible only after a long and tedious off-line computer-aided reconstruction process. Because of extensive research[19,20] and improved technology (eg, faster computers, digital workflow, and new mathematical software tools), the first clinic-ready systems for fused angio/IVUS imaging are being announced.

ANGIOGRAPHY

As mentioned earlier, coronary angiography visualizes the coronary artery tree as a luminal silhouette; for a virtual three-dimensional (3D) impression, the interventionalist must mentally integrate several angiograms at different angulations. This process is not always easy, and

Department of Cardiology, Thoraxcenter, Erasmus Medical Center, P.O. Box 1738, 3000 DR, Rotterdam, The Netherlands
* Corresponding author.
E-mail address: n.bruining@erasmusmc.nl (N. Bruining).

Cardiol Clin 27 (2009) 531–540
doi:10.1016/j.ccl.2009.04.001

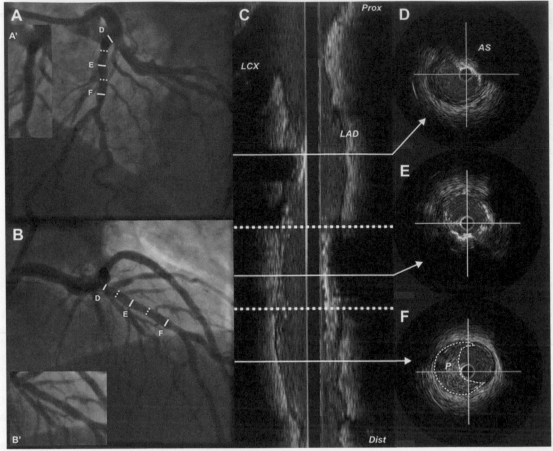

Fig. 1. This clinical case with an implanted bioabsorbable stent in a proximal left anterior descending (LAD) coronary artery shows the advantages of a combined imaging of angiography and IVUS. (*A, B*) Angiographic images of the IVUS images shown in *D* (proximal of the stent), *E* (in-stent), and *F* (distal to the stent). *A'* and *B'* present unblocked views of the angiogram. *C* is a reconstructed longitudinal IVUS view of the stented region (between the two dashed lines) with the distal part at the bottom of the segment and the proximal part at the top. A large calcified area can be seen in *D* but cannot be seen on the angiogram. Furthermore, panel *E* shows that the stent is well positioned to the vessel wall, and *F* shows a large plaque just distal of the stent; neither can be discerned on the angiogram. In such cases the two modalities are complementary. *LAD;* left anterior descendens, *LCX;* left circumflex coronary artery.

establishing a proper diagnosis by means of angiography may be difficult, especially when there are eccentric coronary lesions and bifurcations.

To provide a good impression of diseased coronary segments, the angiograms usually are selected/stopped during a phase of relatively slow motion. Using these still frames, the interventionalist makes the diagnosis, performs measurements (quantitative coronary angiography, QCA[21,22]), and considers the possible treatment options, using visual estimations or QCA measurements to select the appropriate balloon and stent length and diameter.

An advantage of angiography over intravascular imaging techniques is that it can visualize and serve as a road map to the complete coronary artery tree, including very narrow stenoses and

small vessels. Vessel diameters smaller than 1 mm are difficult, if not impossible, to cross with an IVUS catheter.

Given all these considerations, the ideal angiographic visualization would be a computer-reconstructed, true 3D, real-time representation of the coronary artery tree, even if it is only a coronary luminal silhouette. Simultaneous imaging with bi-planar angiography equipment made this visualization possible. A method for using these bi-planar angiograms for modeling a 3D coronary artery tree was described first in 1995.[20] Unfortunately, it has taken almost a decade for this methodology to be adapted (recently the interest in bifurcation stenting seems to be stimulating the integration) and for the technology (eg, computer speed and the interaction between the methods of visualization and the angiography equipment) to be sufficiently advanced for this methodology to be used on-line. An important factor is the digitization of images (standardized through the implementation of the DICOM standard) in the catheterization laboratory workflow.[23]

The constant improvement of the image quality[24] and the recent development of rotational angiography[25] probably will result in an even more standardized and widely accepted use of 3D angiography and 3D computer-reconstructed coronary artery trees.

QUANTITATIVE CORONARY ANGIOGRAPHY

The development of QCA[26,27] was an important step for both procedure guidance and for interventional studies (**Fig. 2**). The availability of a quantitative outcome based on computer-detected contours made QCA the de facto choice as a surrogate end point in many interventional trials,[28,29] and QCA still is used today, despite competition from additional imaging modalities such as IVUS. The technique has been described and validated intensively and is, or can be, incorporated in the modern catheterization laboratory angiography systems from all the major vendors. Also standalone, dedicated analysis stations are available from various vendors for use in both catheterization laboratories and core laboratories. Most of the QCA contour detection algorithms are based on the same basic principles,[30,31] but different QCA software packages can produce different outcomes when using the same patient data.[32]

Therefore, to avoid possible deviations, it is recommended that the same equipment and analysis software be used in longitudinal studies.

Currently, quantitative 3D coronary angiography is becoming popular,[33,34,35] perhaps because the recent developments in bifurcation stenting have resulted in a greater need to analyze complex bifurcation stenosis, which is difficult to judge by 2D angiography alone.[36,37] Bifurcations are very difficult to evaluate on a series of 2D images because of the over-projection of the coronary branches. In this situation, a 3D reconstruction of the coronary lumen would be ideal (**Fig. 3**). To create this reconstruction, all identifiable coronary lumen edges must be detected by a method similar to that used for QCA.

INTRAVASCULAR ULTRASOUND IMAGING

An IVUS examination is performed mostly by retracting the catheter systematically with a device operating at a retraction speed of 0.5 mm/second.[38] Images generated at a speed of 30 frames per second are acquired constantly during the retraction and are stored digitally by the ultrasound console. Modern commercially available IVUS consoles generate a longitudinal view (L-view) in real time during the retraction procedure.[38] This view helps the clinician visualize a comprehensive overview of the investigated segment. Because a retraction procedure takes a considerable amount of valuable catherization laboratory time, most examinations are limited to the region of interest, so the complete coronary

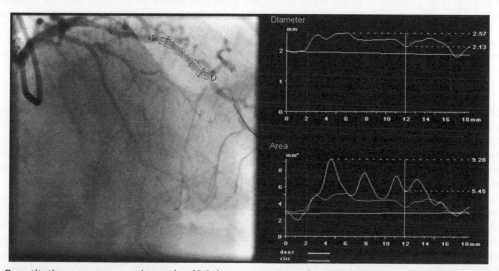

Fig. 2. Quantitative coronary angiography (QCA) measurement. The vessel has been analyzed between the markers P (proximal) and D (distal). The top graph on the right presents the diameters as determined by the QCA software, and the bottom graph presents presumed calculated data, assuming a circular model. These data often are used clinically to select the most appropriate balloon and stent sizes.

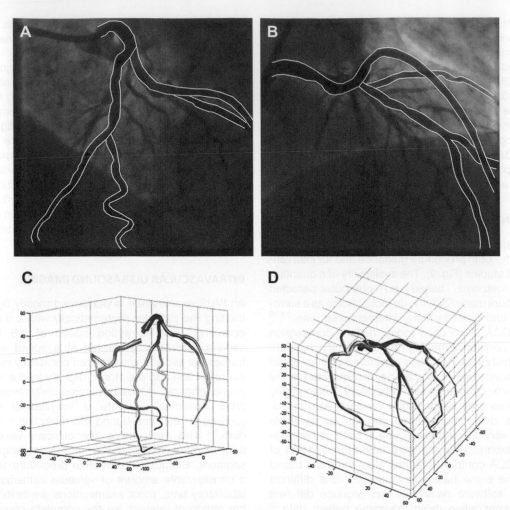

Fig. 3. A possible reconstruction of a coronary artery tree from angiographic data. (*A*, *B*) In at least two perpendicular angiographic projections, all the major vessels and those that should be shown in the final 3D reconstruction must be detected by a semi-automated algorithm. When all these vessels are identified, a 3D reconstruction can be created as can be appreciated in panels *C* and *D*. In this example all three major vessels (the LAD, LCX, and RCA) were extracted. The rotation in panel *C* is approximately that of the projected angiogram in panel *A*, and the rotation in panel *D* is approximately that of panel *B*. For a dynamic reconstruction, all images during one cardiac cycle must undergo the contour detection procedure.

artery tree is not investigated. Furthermore, the L-views are generated without taking the vascular curvature into account, because the IVUS catheter does not acquire 3D spatial information.

One reason that integration of the two imaging modalities has taken so long may be that none of the major angiography equipment vendors have IVUS in their portfolio. Only two major companies currently produce IVUS consoles and catheters: Boston Scientific (BSC, Santa Clara, CA) and Volcano Therapeutics (Santa Clara, CA), and these manufacturers use two different basic IVUS techniques. Boston Scientific produces catheters with single rotating element transducers operating at 40 MHz. Volcano produces catheters with multiple elements in a phased array operating at 20 MHz. Each technique has advantages and disadvantages.[25]. It is expected that catheters operating at higher frequencies will allow an even a more detailed visualization of the coronary vessel wall than possible today.

For the later fusion/integration of both angiography and IVUS, it is important to remember that the IVUS images are acquired constantly during the pullback procedure, without taking into account the possible displacement of the catheter by cardiac motion. These non-gated retractions create a saw-toothed appearance of the vessel wall[39,40] that can hamper the visualization of coronary vessel wall morphology. Not only is the visualization obscured; it also has been reported that the IVUS catheter can shift as much as 5 mm longitudinally because of motion during the cardiac cycle, making later accurate localization and registration difficult.[41] In addition to this longitudinal catheter motion, the heart also rotates around the catheter, as can be seen in IVUS pullback videos. These motion artifacts make accurate registration between the two modalities difficult; therefore, gating of the image acquisition is a necessary step.

Gating of the acquisition image can be performed by on-line ECG gating[40] or by using an image-based retrospectively gated IVUS image selection technique.[42] Volcano uses ECG gating at the time of R-top technique for IVUS-RF data acquisition; Boston Scientific is planning to adopt a similar approach in the near future.

QUANTITATIVE INTRAVASCULAR ULTRASOUND

The development of quantitative intravascular (or intracoronary) ultrasound (QCU) was described first by Li and colleagues,[43] who proposed using a longitudinal reconstructed view of the coronary artery in which, as in QCA, the lumen–intima

interface and the external elastic membrane (used as the outer vessel border) could be detected by computer assistance. The ability of IVUS to visualize the morphology of the coronary vessel wall in high detail has made the QCU technique the de facto standard for evaluating longitudinal progression-regression studies[11,13,43] and was used to evaluate the first generation of bare metal stents and drug-eluting stents.[29] At the Erasmus Medical Center, the authors first apply retrospective gating and then use dedicated vessel analysis software (CURAD B.V., Wijk bij Duurstede, The Netherlands) based on a longitudinal analysis (**Fig. 4**). This software allows the contour data to be exported for later integration with other imaging modalities such as angiography, as described in this article.

IVUS also can be used to evaluate plaque composition,[12,44,45,46] although this evaluation still is subject to large scientific debate. Several companies offer dedicated QCU software.

INTEGRATED IMAGING

The development of integrated angiography and IVUS imaging (**Fig. 5**) can be divided into two

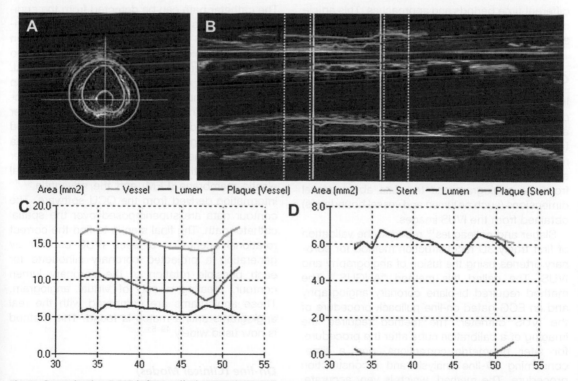

Fig. 4. Quantitative IVUS (often called "quantitative coronary ultrasound," QCU). (*A*) A cross section in which the outer vessel contour is presented in green and the stent contour in blue. (*B*) A stented region (between the thick yellow lines) and an investigated proximal and distal part (each 5 mm of length, between the yellow dashed lines). (*C*) The dimensions of the lumen are shown in red, and , the outer vessel areas are shown in green. The line between shows the area of plaque. (*D*) The lumen and stent area are superimposed. Because the procedure was performed just after stenting, the results are as expected.

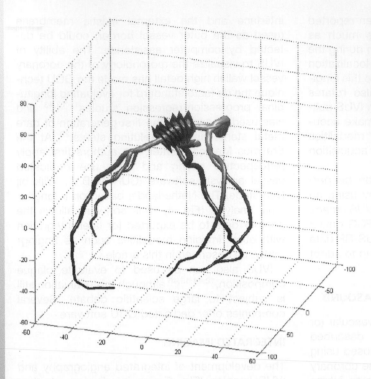

Fig. 5. A 3D reconstructed coronary artery tree is p integrated with the IVUS images. This presentation shows the angle at which the IVUS images were acquired. Spatial information that is not available by IVUS alone can be missed by using longitudinal reconstructed views (L-views) in which it is assumed that the pullback is straight. If these reconstructions could be visualized on-line, combined with the normal 2D angiography and the raw IVUS image data presented in cross section and in an L-view (see **Fig. 1**), the interventionist would have all possible information.

different time periods and approaches. This article distinguishes these time frames and approaches as (1) research modes and (2) clinical modes.

Off-line (Research Modes)

In research, the prime objective of integrated angiography and IVUS is accuracy. Time of acquisition and later reconstruction are not the most important problems to overcome. Most of the described research approaches reconstruct the coronary artery tree by using the spatial information derived from the angiogram and the data about vessel dimensions (such as lumen and vessel boundaries) obtained from the IVUS images.

Slager and colleagues[19] reported the validation of first truely 3D reconstruction method for coronary arteries using the fusion of angiography and IVUS. The called this method "ANGUS." The method required bi-plane coronary angiography and an ECG-gated on-line pullback procedure of the IVUS catheter. The method required the imaging of a calibration cube after the procedure, for later geometric corrections, and a time-consuming off-line analysis and reconstruction procedure. The method, which is very accurate, has been extensively described.[19] The analysis and reconstruction procedure does not use "raw" images but instead uses the results of an extracted catheter path derived from the coronary angiography and the contours detected by IVUS.

The catheter path can be detected from the angiography images only by using sheath-based catheters, such as those manufactured by Boston Scientific. The phased-array catheters of Volcano Therapeutics cannot be used for this method, because these catheters have a free-floating tip that takes an unpredictable path through the coronary artery during the pullback. After the catheter path is detected, the IVUS contours are detected in the IVUS images by identifying the lumen–intima interface and the outer vessel boundary. The latter is detected as the transition between the external elastic membrane (EEM) and the adventitia,[47,48] information derived from the QCU software. The contour data are superimposed over the spatial catheter path. The final step is to find the correct rotational orientation of each IVUS contour by generating a projected coronary silhouette for each possible rotation of the coronary lumen contour, creating a sort of virtual angiogram. These angiograms are compared with the real angiograms until a match is found. This method is now used widely.[49–51]

On-line (Clinical Modes)

The use of a methodology in research often precedes its clinical implementation. When the methodology is developed, optimized, and validated, it progresses from off-line reconstructions to on-line use (with a few minutes allowed for analysis) to, it is hoped, an almost real-time implementation with an easily used interface.

It can be questioned whether the previously described highly accurate research approaches are necessary in the clinic. Are the fancy 3D reconstructions necessary in the catheterization laboratory (**Fig. 5**)? Would such reconstructions improve patient outcomes? Certainly, time-consuming and difficult acquisition procedures will not become popular. The trick is to keep the procedure in the catheterization laboratory as simple as possible. The introduction of the digital catheterization laboratory and the standardization of the images to DICOM have paved the way for the integration of the imaging modalities, although even today this integration is not always straightforward.

Today, several manufacturers of angiography device have adapted one of the imaging monitors at the catheterization laboratory table to allow importation of other DICOM images, such as those from the IVUS consoles. Furthermore, the manufacturers of IVUS devices have investigated means of integrating their consoles into the catheterization laboratory tableside instead of having them on a large and potentially intrusive mobile cart. These adaptations could improve the logistics of side-by-side viewing of the angiogram and IVUS examination (**Fig. 6**).

Although some advanced software tools are under development, they unfortunately will not become commercially available in the near future. Currently, the most common clinical application is a rough correlation of the vessel segment identified on the angiogram with the IVUS examination. After co-registration of the two image sets, performed mostly by using identified side-branches,

a marker is superimposed on the angiogram that corresponds to an IVUS image. This paired presentation if IVUS and angiographic images could help in the interpretation of the images, although it requires some user interaction and is not as accurate as the ANGUS method described previously.[19]

CURRENT AND FUTURE DEVELOPMENTS

The combined fusion imaging and true 3D reconstructions of the coronary artery have been used extensively for research of wall shear stress, vessel curvature, and plaque development.[51–53] This imaging could influence the development of new therapeutic strategies. Additionally, new research and clinical application can be initiated by incorporating magnetic navigation systems[54] to assist complex percutaneous coronary interventions.

Current developments in rotational angiography, minimally invasive MSCT, and noninvasive MRI bring 3D imaging into clinical interventional cardiology. The use of 3D for clinical procedures in cardiology is widely accepted now, but it took a decade to transfer the technology from the research mode to the clinical mode. Coronary angiography probably will change radically, from the traditional 2D format to 3D representation, under the influence of these new technical developments.

It is hoped that the recent introduction of new imaging modalities such as MSCT and optical coherence tomography will encourage the imaging manufactures to design their next generation of imaging systems for a flexible,

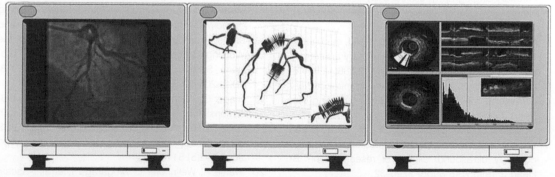

Fig. 6. In the near future a set-up like that shown could give the interventionalist information about the whole coronary artery tree while the patient is on the table. The monitor on the left presents the standard 2D angiography (or, in the future, rotational angiography acquisitions). The monitor on the right presents the intracoronary ultrasound data, possibly both live and a quantitative analysis that might include information about plaque composition (here derived using echogenicity analysis). 3D reconstructions and analysis could be presented on the middle monitor. In this example two vessels have been examined by IVUS, and the regions where the images were acquired are identified by fusing the 3D reconstructed angiography data with the IVUS data superimposed on it.

multimodality imaging environment. Although some of the modalities have been presented as the only imaging method needed in the catheterization laboratory, most of the modalities currently in use are not competitors but rather are complementary.

SUMMARY

Multimodality imaging will be increasingly important in the evaluation of patients who have coronary artery disease and in the evaluation of new interventional therapies. Combined and integrated IVUS-angiography imaging has proved a valuable complement to the standard imaging repertoire in the catheterization laboratory. The manufacturers of both X-ray angiography and IVUS systems must make this integration clinically acceptable with a seamless workflow. It is hoped that this final integration of technology will be addressed in the near future.

REFERENCES

1. Sones FM Jr. Cine-coronary arteriography. Ohio Med 1962;58:1018–9.
2. St. Goar FG, Pinto FJ, Alderman EL, et al. Intravascular ultrasound imaging of angiographically normal coronary arteries: an in vivo comparison with quantitative angiography. J Am Coll Cardiol 1991;18(4):952–8.
3. De Scheerder I, De Man F, Herregods MC, et al. Intravascular ultrasound versus angiography for measurement of luminal diameters in normal and diseased coronary arteries. Am Heart J 1994;127(2):243–51.
4. White CJ, Ramee SR, Collins TJ, et al. Ambiguous coronary angiography: clinical utility of intravascular ultrasound. Cathet Cardiovasc Diagn 1992;26(3):200–3.
5. Fitzgerald PJ, St. Goar FG, Connolly AJ, et al. Intravascular ultrasound imaging of coronary arteries. Is three layers the norm? Circulation 1992;86(1):154–8.
6. Lee DY, Eigler N, Luo H, et al. Effect of intracoronary ultrasound imaging on clinical decision making. Am Heart J 1995;129(6):1084–93.
7. Di Mario C, von Birgelen C, Prati F, et al. Three dimensional reconstruction of cross sectional intracoronary ultrasound: clinical or research tool? Br Heart J 1995;73(5 Suppl 2):26–32.
8. Mudra H, Klauss V, Blasini R, et al. Ultrasound guidance of Palmaz-Schatz intracoronary stenting with a combined intravascular ultrasound balloon catheter. Circulation 1994;90(3):1252–61.
9. Tobis J, Azarbal B, Slavin L. Assessment of intermediate severity coronary lesions in the catheterization laboratory. J Am Coll Cardiol 2007;49(8):839–48.
10. Pasterkamp G, Mali WP, Borst C. Application of intravascular ultrasound in remodelling studies. Semin Interv Cardiol 1997;2(1):11–8.
11. Nissen SE, Tsunoda T, Tuzcu EM, et al. Effect of recombinant ApoA-I Milano on coronary atherosclerosis in patients with acute coronary syndromes: a randomized controlled trial. JAMA 2003;290(17):2292–300.
12. Serruys PW, Garcia-Garcia HM, Buszman P, et al. Effects of the direct lipoprotein-associated phospholipase A(2) inhibitor darapladib on human coronary atherosclerotic plaque. Circulation 2008;118(11):1172–82.
13. Rodriguez-Granillo GA, de Winter S, Bruining N, et al. Effect of perindopril on coronary remodelling: insights from a multicentre, randomized study. Eur Heart J 2007;28(19):2326–31.
14. Ormiston JA, Serruys PW, Regar E, et al. A bioabsorbable everolimus-eluting coronary stent system for patients with single de-novo coronary artery lesions (ABSORB): a prospective open-label trial. Lancet 2008;371(9616):899–907.
15. Grube E, Gerckens U, Buellesfeld L, et al. Images in cardiovascular medicine. Intracoronary imaging with optical coherence tomography: a new high-resolution technology providing striking visualization in the coronary artery. Circulation 2002;106(18):2409–10.
16. Achenbach S, Ropers D, Hoffmann U, et al. Assessment of coronary remodeling in stenotic and nonstenotic coronary atherosclerotic lesions by multidetector spiral computed tomography. J Am Coll Cardiol 2004;43(5):842–7.
17. Nieman K, Oudkerk M, Rensing BJ, et al. Coronary angiography with multi-slice computed tomography. Lancet 2001;357(9256):599–603.
18. Di Mario C, Gorge G, Peters R, et al. Clinical application and image interpretation in intracoronary ultrasound. Study Group on Intracoronary Imaging of the Working Group of Coronary Circulation and of the Subgroup on Intravascular Ultrasound of the Working Group of Echocardiography of the European Society of Cardiology. Eur Heart J 1998;19(2):207–29.
19. Slager CJ, Wentzel JJ, Schuurbiers JC, et al. True 3-dimensional reconstruction of coronary arteries in patients by fusion of angiography and IVUS (ANGUS) and its quantitative validation. Circulation 2000;102(5):511–6.
20. Wahle A, Wellnhofer E, Mugaragu I, et al. Assessment of diffuse coronary artery disease by quantitative analysis of coronary morphology based upon 3-D reconstruction from biplane angiograms. IEEE Trans Med Imaging 1995;14(2):230–41.
21. Serruys PW, Reiber JH, Wijns W, et al. Assessment of percutaneous transluminal coronary angioplasty by quantitative coronary angiography: diameter

versus densitometric area measurements. Am J Cardiol 1984;54(6):482–8.

22. Reiber JH, Serruys PW, Kooijman CJ, et al. Assessment of short-, medium-, and long-term variations in arterial dimensions from computer-assisted quantitation of coronary cineangiograms. Circulation 1985;71(2):280–8.

23. Bidgood WD Jr, Horii SC. Introduction to the ACR-NEMA DICOM standard. Radiographics 1992; 12(2):345–55.

24. Noumeir R. Benefits of the DICOM structured report. J Digit Imaging 2006;19(4):295–306.

25. Suselbeck T, Latsch A, von Furstenberg M, et al. [Expansion of the Multilink-Tristar stent after direct implantation and predilatation: comparison of clinical, angiography and intravascular ultrasound parameters]. Z Kardiol 2002;91(6):487–92 [in German].

26. Reiber JH, van Eldik-Helleman P, Visser-Akkerman N, et al. Variabilities in measurement of coronary arterial dimensions resulting from variations in cineframe selection. Cathet Cardiovasc Diagn 1988;14(4):221–8.

27. Serruys PW, Luijten HE, Beatt KJ, et al. Incidence of restenosis after successful coronary angioplasty: a time-related phenomenon. A quantitative angiographic study in 342 consecutive patients at 1, 2, 3, and 4 months. Circulation 1988;77(2): 361–71.

28. Foley DP, Melkert R, Umans VA, et al. Differences in restenosis propensity of devices for transluminal coronary intervention. A quantitative angiographic comparison of balloon angioplasty, directional atherectomy, stent implantation and excimer laser angioplasty. CARPORT, MERCATOR, MARCATOR, PARK, and BENESTENT Trial Groups. Eur Heart J 1995; 16(10):1331–46.

29. Serruys PW, de Jaegere P, Kiemeneij F, et al. A comparison of balloon-expandable-stent implantation with balloon angioplasty in patients with coronary artery disease. Benestent Study Group. N Engl J Med 1994;331(8):489–95.

30. Reiber JH, Kooijman CJ, Slager CJ, et al. Coronary artery dimensions from cineangiograms methodology and validation of a computer-assisted analysis procedure. IEEE Trans Med Imaging 1984;3(3): 131–41.

31. Reiber JH, van der Zwet PM, Koning G, et al. Accuracy and precision of quantitative digital coronary arteriography: observer-, short-, and medium-term variabilities. Cathet Cardiovasc Diagn 1993;28(3): 187–98.

32. Keane D, Haase J, Slager CJ, et al. Comparative validation of quantitative coronary angiography systems. Results and implications from a multicenter study using a standardized approach. Circulation 1995;91(8):2174–83.

33. Agostoni P, Biondi-Zoccai G, Van Langenhove G, et al. Comparison of assessment of native coronary arteries by standard versus three-dimensional coronary angiography. Am J Cardiol 2008;102(3):272–9.

34. Ramcharitar S, Daeman J, Patterson M, et al. First direct in vivo comparison of two commercially available three-dimensional quantitative coronary angiography systems. Catheter Cardiovasc Interv 2008;71(1):44–50.

35. Wahle A, Prause PM, DeJong SC, et al. Geometrically correct 3-D reconstruction of intravascular ultrasound images by fusion with biplane angiography—methods and validation. IEEE Trans Med Imaging 1999;18(8):686–99.

36. Latib A, Colombo A, Sangiorgi G. Bifurcation stenting: current strategies and new devices. Heart (British Cardiac Society) 2009;95(6):495–504.

37. Adriaenssens T, Byrne RA, Dibra A, et al. Culotte stenting technique in coronary bifurcation disease: angiographic follow-up using dedicated quantitative coronary angiographic analysis and 12 month clinical outcomes. Eur Heart J 2008;29(23):2868–76.

38. Mintz GS, Nissen SE, Anderson WD, et al. American college of cardiology clinical expert consensus document on standards for acquisition, measurement and reporting of intravascular ultrasound studies (ivus). a report of the american college of cardiology task force on clinical expert consensus documents. J Am Coll Cardiol 2001;37(5):1478–92.

39. Bruining N, von Birgelen C, de Feyter PJ, et al. ECG-gated versus nongated three-dimensional intracoronary ultrasound analysis: implications for volumetric measurements. Cathet Cardiovasc Diagn 1998; 43(3):254–60.

40. von Birgelen C, de Vrey EA, Mintz GS, et al. ECG-gated three-dimensional intravascular ultrasound: feasibility and reproducibility of the automated analysis of coronary lumen and atherosclerotic plaque dimensions in humans. Circulation 1997;96(9): 2944–52.

41. Arbab-Zadeh A, DeMaria AN, Penny WF, et al. Axial movement of the intravascular ultrasound probe during the cardiac cycle: implications for three-dimensional reconstruction and measurements of coronary dimensions. Am Heart J 1999;138(5 Pt 1): 865–72.

42. De Winter SA, Hamers R, Degertekin M, et al. Retrospective image-based gating of intracoronary ultrasound images for improved quantitative analysis: the Intelligate method. Catheter Cardiovasc Interv 2004;61(1):84–94.

43. Li W, von Birgelen C, Di Mario C, et al. Semi-automated contour detection for volumetric quantification of intracoronary ultrasound. Comput Cardiol 1994;21:277–80.

44. Nissen SE. Application of intravascular ultrasound to characterize coronary artery disease and assess the

progression or regression of atherosclerosis. Am J Cardiol 2002;89(4A):24B–31.

45. Bruining N, Verheye S, Knaapen M, et al. Three-dimensional and quantitative analysis of atherosclerotic plaque composition by automated differential echogenicity. Catheter Cardiovasc Interv 2007; 70(7):968–78.

46. Nair A, Kuban BD, Tuzcu EM, et al. Coronary plaque classification with intravascular ultrasound radiofrequency data analysis. Circulation 2002;106(17): 2200–6.

47. Wenguang L, Gussenhoven WJ, Zhong Y, et al. Validation of quantitative analysis of intravascular ultrasound images. Int J Cardiovasc Imaging 1991; 6(3–4):247–53.

48. Hamers R, Bruining N, Knook M, et al. A novel approach to quantitative analysis of intravascular ultrasound images. Comput Cardiol 2001;28:589–92.

49. Wahle A, Prause GP, von Birgelen C, et al. Fusion of angiography and intravascular ultrasound in vivo: establishing the absolute 3-D frame orientation. IEEE Trans Biomed Eng 1999;46(10):1176–80.

50. Bourantas CV, Kourtis IC, Plissiti ME, et al. A method for 3D reconstruction of coronary arteries using biplane angiography and intravascular ultrasound images. Comput Med Imaging Graph 2005;29(8): 597–606.

51. Wahle A, Lopez JJ, Olszewski ME, et al. Plaque development, vessel curvature, and wall shear stress in coronary arteries assessed by X-ray angiography and intravascular ultrasound. Med Image Anal 2006;10(4):615–31.

52. Slager CJ, Wentzel JJ, Gijsen FJ, et al. The role of shear stress in the destabilization of vulnerable plaques and related therapeutic implications. Nature 2005;2(9):456–64.

53. Slager CJ, Wentzel JJ, Gijsen FJ, et al. The role of shear stress in the generation of rupture-prone vulnerable plaques. Nature 2005;2(8):401–7.

54. Ramcharitar S, van Geuns RJ, Patterson M, et al. A randomized comparison of the magnetic navigation system versus conventional percutaneous coronary intervention. Catheter Cardiovasc Interv 2008; 72(6):761–70.

The Future Cardiac Catheterization Laboratory

S. James Chen, PhD*, Adam R. Hansgen, BS, John D. Carroll, MD

KEYWORDS

- Image fusion • Robot-assisted intervention
- Multimodality fusion • Holographic rendering
- Pathway tortuosity • Coronary artery deformation

Although X-ray angiography has been widely accepted and used as a real-time imaging modality, its traditional format is still limited by its two-dimensional (2D) representation of three-dimensional (3D) structures and the consequent imaging artifacts that impair optimal visualization. More than 50 years after the performance of first coronary angiogram, the basic principle of coronary angiography has not changed, even with the introduction of modern X-ray imaging system. Recognition of these limitations has resulted in the development of 3D imaging techniques designed to address specifically the weaknesses of traditional angiographic techniques. Recent technical endeavors focus mainly on reduction of the X-ray dose, 3D coronary reconstruction and quantitative analysis, optimal viewing strategy, and enhancement of stent visualization. The final representation, however, is still limited to the traditional 2D display format, which is inherently flawed for helping the interventionist appreciate the patient's true 3D anatomy and interaction with the implanted device in vivo.

Recently, the focus in heart disease research and treatment has been expanded from coronary artery disease (CAD) to structural heart disease (SHD). The categories of SHD include hemodynamic and electrophysiologic abnormalities of any of the four cardiac chambers, any of the four heart valves, and the presence of congenital or acquired defects between heart chambers and the great vessels. SHD affects approximately 5 million people in the United States, and approximately 1 million of those cases require surgical intervention each year. The development of novel interventional therapies for SHD has followed the recognition that growing population of patients who have SHD are being suboptimally treated with palliative medication-based therapy; open heart surgery is the major surgical option. Therefore innovative approaches in visualization are more important and urgent in SHD treatment than CAD treatment to facilitate diagnosis, plan therapy, to provide image-guidance of interventions, to clarify anatomical and pathophysiological issues, and to quantify device–anatomy interactions.

The physicians who perform image-guided interventions in CAD or SHD do not have the advantage of direct observation of the therapeutic target that surgeons often enjoy. These issues are compounded for most cardiologists by their limited training and experience in navigation and visual-spatial skills in the complex 3D spatial relationships of the whole heart and novel device/anatomy fitting. Preprocedural planning for interventions typically uses the 2D imaging of echocardiography and angiography. SHD interventions usually are performed with fluoroscopic image guidance with a variable use of 2D ultrasound. During the last 5 years, a quest has begun to modify existing modalities or to develop other imaging modalities to guide interventions in SHD and cardiac electrophysiological procedures. This transition is driven by the frequent inability to visualize the target of the intervention (valves, chamber defects, heart muscle, and cardiac conduction tissue) by fluoroscopy and by the

Division of Cardiology, Department of Medicine, University of Colorado Denver, Leprino Office Building, Mail Stop B132, 12401 East 17th Avenue, Aurora, CO 80045, USA
* Corresponding author.
E-mail address: james.chen@ucdenver.edu (S.J. Chen).

Cardiol Clin 27 (2009) 541–548
doi:10.1016/j.ccl.2009.04.003
0733-8651/09/$ – see front matter © 2009 Elsevier Inc. All rights reserved.

need for real-time anatomy-based imaging. The community is starting to understand that current diagnostic imaging and image-guidance technology developed for CAD intervention is not completely optimal (**Fig. 1**A and B) and is far from adequate for SHD interventions.

CAD and SHD are increasingly examined and visualized by anatomically based imaging such as cardiac MRI, multidetector computer tomography (MDCT), and high-quality 2D or 3D echocardiography as shown in **Fig. 1**C. When patients who have SHD undergo interventions, the cardiac imaging studies may be displayed on a computer screen for static road mapping to display visually the pathway to the target and the target itself. These volumetric data sets from MDCT or MR angiography, however, are not incorporated into cardiac catheterization laboratory (CCL) as an on-line mechanism for guiding the deployment and placement of an intracoronary or intracardiac device to the targeted location. Additionally, the current suboptimal assessment of the morphology of heart disease and surrounding structures leads

to the design of devices for CAD or SHD that are not necessarily the best for complex coronary lesions and cardiac defects with more variable and complex shapes, orientations, and sizes that may change dynamically during the cardiac cycle. Therefore improved and even customized stent and closure devices are needed, and the dimensions and shape of these devices should be calculated precisely from cardiac imaging modalities to fit the patient-specific coronary stenosis or morphologic defect.

As new CAD and SHD interventions are developed, traditional 2D visualization should be complemented by (or fused with) other modalities that display complementary features and emphasize physicality and true 3D visualization as basic visualization tools in the next generation of cardiac catherization laboratories. Additionally, robot-assisted catheter navigation and tracking can be incorporated in conjunction with the hybrid 3D and 4D anatomic imaging for optimal selection, efficient delivery, and accurate placement of therapeutic devices. The typical cardiac

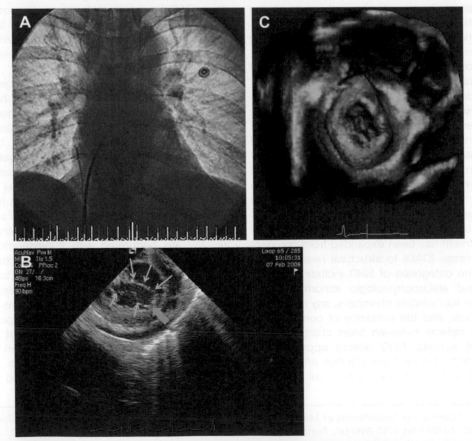

Fig. 1. (A) The fluoroscopic image with the intracardiac echocardiography (ICE) probe (*lower left corner*) to assist SHD intervention. (B) The 2D real-time ICE image showing the defect of mitral valve (*blue arrow*) and leaflets (*orange arrows*). (C) The live 3D TEE image of the mitral valve as seen from the top.

catheterization laboratory of the future, equipped with modern multiple imaging modalities, advanced 3D quantitative analysis utilities, real-time navigation, and truly 3D rendering equipment, is illustrated in **Fig. 2** and is discussed in detail in the following sections.

ADVANCED THREE-DIMENSIONAL QUANTITATIVE ANALYSIS

Difficult or failed delivery of stents to a target area during percutaneous coronary interventions (PCI) may result from excessive vessel tortuosity and the take-off angle of branching vessel in the deivery pathway. Similarly, it would be more challenging to perform intervention for mitral valve repair if the delivery pathway involves multiple components of the heart such as the superior vena cava, the right atrium, left atrium, and the left ventricle. With the ability to create patient-specific 3D anatomy of the heart (ie, the coronary arterial tree, great vessels, and heart chamber), the pathway to the target region, the size of stenotic lesion, and the shape of defect can be assessed and quantified to facilitate optimal patient selection and adequate fitting of therapeutic device (eg, guide-wire, catheter, stent, and occluder) for CAD or SHD intervention.

If a library of end-diastolic and end-systolic vessel curvature values (**Fig. 3**) can be constructed for patients undergoing PCI, it will represent the retrospective cataloging experience with outcomes of PCI accompanied with various degrees of vessel tortuosity. The results will be displayed according to the vessel involved and the composite pathway that must be traversed to the target lesion. Curvature values corresponding to unsuccessful or difficult delivery (ie, PCI outcome experience) will be highlighted and used to derive a predictive model from which the likelihood of success in device delivery will be calculated by using the curvature values extracted from the current patient's 3D coronary arteries and will be presented to clinician for optimal selection of intracoronary devices during intervention.

The type, size, location, and number of defects in SHD vary widely from heart to heart. The attention to geometrical features and proximity to surrounding structures will help in assessing a patient's suitability for device closure and in designing more efficient and appropriate devices. Similar to the creation of a coronary library, the database of various patient-specific heart models will be generated from volumetric data sets acquired from either MDCT or MRI. With the 3D heart models, various geometrical features of heart anatomy can be categorized such as (1) estimates of length and tortuosity associated with different pathways from the inferior vena cava, superior vena cava, aorta, and pulmonary artery to different chambers (**Fig. 4**A), (2) the chamber's or defect's dimensions, including thickness, shape, and rim size, as shown in **Fig. 4**B, (3) dynamic changes in the defect over time, and (4) spatial relationships among the major surrounding structures, including distance and orientation. With the use of the anatomic libraries of coronary arteries and hearts, the disease characterization of any patient can be evaluated quickly to direct safer and more efficient treatment based on data regarding previous outcomes, efficacy, and device performance.

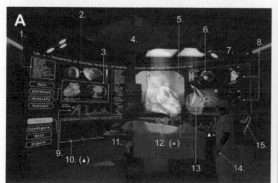 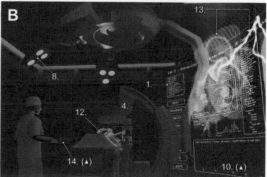

Fig. 2. (*A*) Front and (*B*) lateral views of the configuration of the future cardiac catheterization laboratory. The major components are an X-ray imaging system, an advanced 3D quantitative analysis module, structural and functional imaging modalities, robot-assisted manipulator and navigation, electrophysiology monitoring system, and a true 3D rendering device. (1) Patient History, (2) Functional PET/fMR, (3) CT/MR Imaging, (4) X-ray Imaging System, (5) X-ray Fluoroscopic Display, (6) Structural Echo Imaging, (7) Video Camera, (8) Functional Echo Imaging, (9) Advanced Quantitative Coronary/Stent Analysis, (10) Display of Physician's Motion Tracking Gloves, (11) Patient Table, (12) Robot Manipulator and Navigation controlled by Motion Tracking Gloves, (13) Multi-Modality Fusion and Holographic True 3D Rendering, (14) Motion Tracking Glove, (15) Advanced Pathway Analysis.

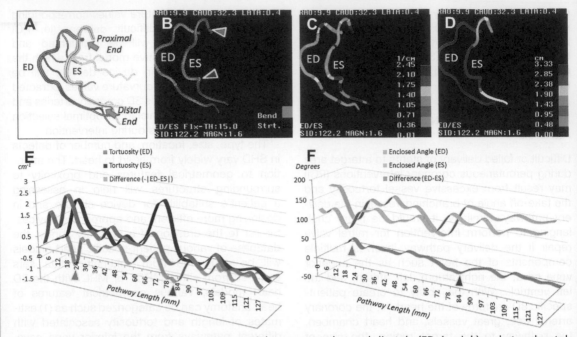

Fig. 3. (*A*) The 3D models of right coronary arterial trees created at end-diastole (ED, in pink) and at end-systole (ES, in yellow) in which the pathways (*blue curves*) from the ostium to the atrioventricular node branch are selected for analysis. (*B*) The points of bending flexion (*red triangle*) and stretching flexion (*blue triangle*) (>15°) are identified. (*C*) The tortuosity estimates for each pathway and (*D*) the translational movement between the two pathways are calculated and displayed in color. In the detailed representations of (*E*) tortuosity and (*F*) the flexion angle for each pathway and their difference, the two prominent flexion points are indicated by the blue and red triangles.

MULTIMODALITY FUSION

Medical diagnoses commonly rely on assessment of both the functional status and the anatomic condition of the patient. The emergence of MDCT and MRI of anatomic structures changes the paradigm. The volumetric 3D nature of these images potentially can be used for the subsequent planning and execution of invasive procedures that typically involve a therapeutic intervention.

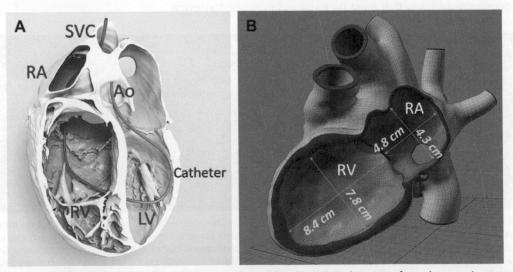

Fig. 4. (*A*) A highly theoretical and complex pathway for aortic valve repair that starts from the superior vena cava (SVC), travels through right atrium (RA) and right ventricle (RV), and enters to the left ventricle (LV) to approach the aorta root (Ao). (*B*) A typical evaluation of the length and width in each individual right atrium (RA) and right ventricle (RV) chamber.

In a clinical setting, in vivo measurement of organ physiology, tissue metabolism, tissue perfusion, and other biologic functions can be performed with radionuclide-tracer techniques such as positron emission tomography (PET) and single-photon emission computed tomography (SPECT). Radionuclide imaging, however, has relatively poor spatial resolution, often is photon starved, and can lack the anatomic cues needed to localize or stage the disease. Recently introduced real-time or live 3D transesophageal echocardiography (TEE)[1,2] allows online accurate assessment of cardiac structures (see **Fig. 1C**). This new technique provides improved anatomic definition and novel views of complex cardiac abnormalities in valve anatomy. Such a real-time imaging system has been used widely to guide difficult SHD interventions including complex atrial septum defect and patent foramen ovale closure, mitral balloon valvotomy, mitral repair using the Evalve clip, and alcohol septal ablation of obstructive hypertrophic cardiomyopathy.[3–5]

With the advent of dual-modality systems, separate detectors for X-ray and PET or SPECT radionuclide imaging are integrated on a common gantry to simplify patient handling, data acquisition, and co-registration of the CT and radionuclide image data. Although hybrid systems produce images that are intrinsically registered because the scans are obtained immediately after one another with the patient in the same position, an alignment process still is needed to improve the registration error caused by cardiac or respiratory motion in cardiac or abdomen imaging. The use such system has

distinct benefits in cardiac applications, allowing physician to do a complete cardiology work-up, performing both CT angiography to detect occlusion and PET to evaluate viability and perfusion. The hybrid imaging system allows the simultaneous acquisition of images on the same machine and provides the most accurate anatomical fusion within about 20 minutes. In cardiac PET/CT, this ability to detect infarcts may increase the versatility and integrative potential of the PET and CT study components of the study.[6,7]

All these clinically available modalities can be characterized by their imaging resolutions, anatomic and functional visibilities, and real-time imaging capability (**Fig. 5**). Although MDCT and MRI are classified as high-resolution imaging modalities, the images currently cannot be acquired in real time. On the other hand, X-ray fluoroscopic imaging is limited to the illustration of soft tissue–based structures such as myocardium but is excellent for real-time display of an intracardiac or intracoronary catheter during interventions. The motion patterns of heart chambers and valves can be captured well by 2D/3D echocardiography but lack the required details in anatomic structure because of the low signal-to-noise ratio. Therefore the complementary features of these imaging modalities need to be incorporated via an advanced fusion process that accounts for differences among the integrated modalities in spatial and temporal resolutions, cardiac and respiratory motions, and morphology and anatomic landmarks.

The current SHD intervention assisted by intra-cardiac echocardiography (ICE) imaging generally

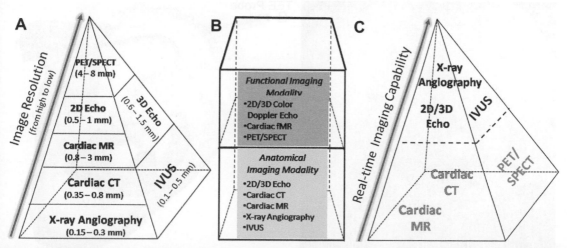

Fig. 5. (A) The classification of various resolutions, ranging from high to low, in different imaging modalities. (B) The anatomically and functionally based dimensions commonly used clinically. (C) Comparisons of the characteristics of various imaging modalities where the imaging modality at the top of pyramid is used as real-time guidance during the therapeutic procedure, and the imaging modality at the bottom of pyramid is commonly adopted for off-line–based diagnostic study.

requires adequate location and orientation of the ICE probe inside the right atrium so that the defect and the surrounding structures can be visualized adequately. This technique generally requires a long learning curve. Also, whether the imaging device is placed at the best location is never known with certainty, and the procedural time can be prolonged dramatically if multiple views of a single target are required or if multiple therapeutic targets are present. With multimodality fusion between live fluoroscopy and MDCT, the ICE probe can be tracked and adjusted in real time to the patient-specific chamber anatomy, as shown in **Fig. 6**A. **Fig. 6**B shows another example of imaging fusion based on MDCT and 3D TEE, in which the interaction between the catheter the pathway inside heart chamber can be monitored globally using registered MDCT, and the orientation and position of catheter tip can be tracked locally in real time using the 3D TEE imaging system.

NAVIGATION AND TRUE THREE-DIMENSIONAL RENDERING

Lacking complete anatomic roadmaps and direct observation of the therapeutic target, physicians who perform image-guided interventions can rely only on fluoroscopic images assisted with 2D or 3D echocardiography to advance a catheter or therapeutic devices to the desired position by using a repeated trial-and-error approach. If the location and orientation of the catheter could be tracked in a real-time navigation system, the therapeutic device (eg, a bifurcation stent or occluder) could

be deployed and placed at the target location more quickly and more effectively than with conventional methods. In addition, the X-ray exposure and dosage of contrast agent can be reduced dramatically with the assistance of the navigation system.

Typically, a navigation system consists of a 3D tracking system and a 3D multi-modality imaging system. The 3D tracking system has two major components, a sensor unit and an emitter unit. These units can use optical, magnetic, radio, or microwave signals. The 3D multimodality imaging system generates visual information based on available imaging modalities such as anatomically based MDCT or MR images or functionally based PET or SPECT data.

Before the tracking process is initiated, the 3D multimodality-based data set needs to be registered with the patient's location and orientation on the table during the intervention. In an intervention-based navigation, the emitter unit is located at the tip of a catheter. The location of the catheter tip must be matched and displayed within the patient's anatomy based on the registered 3D multimodality data set. Navigation systems linked to interventions must have accurate, perfectly registered data sets that compensate for cardiac and respiratory motion to correlate with the patient's physical condition. Additionally, a feedback mechanism (eg, a real-time imaging modality such as fluoroscopy or 2D/3D echocardiography) is required to monitor periodically and to adjust the current location and orientation of the tracking object.

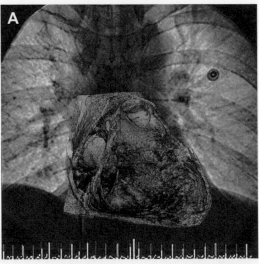

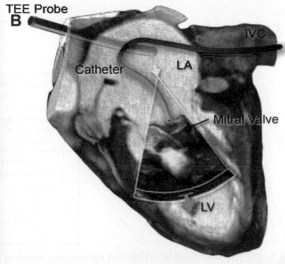

Fig. 6. (*A*) The fusion between MDCT and live fluoroscopy to guide SHD intervention allows the location of the ICE probe inside the chambers to be tracked clearly based on the superimposed MDCT. (*B*) The fusion between MDCT and live 3D TEE illustrating the spatial relationship of the mitral valve, the device catheter, and the surrounding anatomy. LA, left atrium; LV, left ventricle.

It is apparent that a true 3D display allows more intuitive and thus more rapid assessment of the spatial relationships of catheters in 3D spaces than possible with conventional 2D imaging and visualization modalities. For in-room real-time visual guidance during the coronary and intracardiac intervention, the hybrid images resulting from the multimodality fusion process and the geometrical representation of the object being tracked in a navigation system need to be rendered in a truly 3D display based on holographic imaging.

The current 3D display incorporates a variety of techniques such as volumetric, stereoscopic, multiview, and electro-holographic projection.[8] Generally, multiplanar and multiview displays have very different designs. Multiplanar displays have a volumetric format that generates images actually occupying a region in space. A typical volumetric display may provide imagery of 1 to more than 100 million voxels. Generally multiplanar displays operate by projecting patterned light onto seven or eight rotating, reciprocating surfaces undergoing periodic motion. Multiview displays, on the other hand, project views to observers situated in one or more locations. Increasing the number of views in a multiview display increases the accuracy of the projected light field. One of the multiview technologies is holographic imaging,[9,10] in which the motions of an array of micro-mirrors are controlled by computer to fragmentize and redirect an array of laser rays to make 3D holographic pictures of anatomic features.[11]

ROBOT-ASSISTED INTERVENTIONS BASED ON AN ACTIVE CATHETER

Robot-assisted surgery moves minimally invasive surgery to a new level. Patients potentially have less pain and scarring, reduced bleeding, and faster recovery times. At present the most common robot-assisted oprations include cardiovascular and thoracic procedures, gynecology procedures, urology procedures, and gastrointestinal procedures. Unlike conventional laparoscopic surgery, the robotic system provides unprecedented, highly magnified, 3D views of the operating field, eliminates tremors in the surgeon's hand movements, and allows greater freedom of motion for instruments. The use of robots for minimally invasive interventions in the operating room has been investigated closely for preoperative planning and surgery.[12–18]

The basic robot-assisted system for coronary or intracardiac intervention will involve a robotic manipulator with a controllable catheter (or active catheter)[19–21] under the direction and guidance of an interventionist. The tip of the active catheter will be tracked in real time using a navigation system with a true 3D rendering display to provide information on the location and orientation of the catheter to determine the additional distance of insertion or the rotational movement required for the robot and the necessary bending angle for the active catheter. The use of a robotic-assisted system improved visualization and precision that are crucial for the interventionist working in close proximity and limited space inside the heart or coronary artery.

Interventional cardiologists are at risk from radiation exposure because of lengthy procedures performed under X-ray radiations. A clinician performs several thousand such procedures during his/her lifetime, leading to a substantial accumulation of or exposure to radiation. With robot-assisted guidance, the catheter can be advanced autonomously from the point of entry to the site of stenosis in a coronary artery or to the site of a septal defect in a cardiac chamber. The clinician is spared the exposure to harmful radiation from the X-rays used for imaging, and the therapeutic device is delivered more rapidly and effectively than with conventional approach.

SUMMARY

The interventional field moves forward by the invention of new devices, drugs, and biologic agents and also through the refinements and breakthroughs in imaging guidance that enable the interventionist to perform these new treatments. Unlike coronary interventions that use an over-the-wire pathway for devices in a confined branching vascular tree, many new interventions require 3D visualization for navigation in the open space of cardiac chambers. The combination of state-of-the-art robot-assisted intervention, multimodality fusion, true 3D rendering, advanced navigation systems, and innovative therapy should offer patients the best chance for survival and improved quality of life.

REFERENCES

1. Houck RC, Cooke JE, Gill EA. Live 3D echocardiography: a replacement for traditional 2D echocardiography? AJR 2006;187:1092–106.
2. Hung J, Lang R, Flachskampf F, et al. 3D echocardiography: a review of the current status and future directions. J Am Soc Echocardiogr 2007;20(3): 213–33.

3. Kim M, Klein A, Carroll JD. Transcatheter closure of intracardiac defects in adult. J Interv Cardiol 2007; 20(6):524–45.

4. Garcia JA, Eng MH, Wink O, et al. Image guidance of percutaneous coronary and structural heart disease interventions using a computed tomography and fluoroscopic integration. Vasc Dis Manag 2007; 4(3):89–97.

5. Eng M, Salcedo E, Quaife R, et al. Real-time 3-dimensional percutaneous structural heart disease interventions. J Am Coll Cardiol, submitted.

6. Holz A, Lautamaki R, Sasano T, et al. Expanding the versatility of cardiac PET/CT: feasibility of delayed contrast enhancement CT for infarct detection in a porcine model. J Nucl Med 2009;50(2):259–65.

7. Di Carli MF, Dorbala S, Meserve J, et al. Clinical myocardial perfusion PET/CT. J Nucl Med 2007;48: 783–93.

8. Favalora GE. Volumetric 3D displays and application infrastructure. Computer 2005;38(8):37–44.

9. Huebschman M, Munjuluri B, Garner HR. Dynamic holographic 3-D image projection. Opt Express 2003;11(5):437–45.

10. Bove VM Jr., Plesniaka WJ, Quentmeyera T, et al. Real-time holographic video images with commodity PC hardware. San Jose, CA. Proc. SPIE 2005;5664: 255–62.

11. Chun W, Napoli J, Cossairt OS, et al. Spatial 3-D infrastructure: display-independent software framework, high-speed rendering electronics, and several new displays. Proceedings of the SPIE 2005;5664: 302–12.

12. Falk V, Diegeler A, Walther T, et al. Endoscopic coronary artery bypass grafting on the beating heart using a computer enhanced telemanipulation system. Heart Surg Forum 1999;2:199–205.

13. Menon M, Tewari A. Robotic radical prostatectomy and the Vattikuti Urology Institute technique: an interim analysis of results and technical points. Urology 2003;61:15–20.

14. Ostlie DJ, Miller KA, Woods RK, et al. Single cannula technique and robotic telescopic assistance in infants and children who require laparoscopic Nissen fundoplication. J Pediatr Surg 2003;38(1): 111–5.

15. Reichenspurner H, Boehm DH, Welz A, et al. 3D-video- and robot-assisted port access mitral valve surgery. Ann Thorac Surg 1998;1(2):104–6.

16. Ashton RC, Connery CP, Swistel DG, et al. Robot-assisted lobectomy. J Thorac Cardiovasc Surg 2003;126(1):292–3.

17. Bodner J, Wykypiel H, Greiner A, et al. Early experience with robot-assisted surgery for mediastinal masses. Ann Thorac Surg 2004;78:259–65.

18. Delingette H, Pennec X, Soler L, et al. Computational models for image-guided robot-assisted and simulated medical interventions. Proceedings of the IEEE 2006;94(9):1678–88.

19. Park KT, Esashi M. A multilink active catheter with polyimide-based integrated CMOS interface circuits. J Microelectromech Syst 1999;8(4):349–57.

20. Araki T, Aoki S, Ishigame K, et al. MR-guided intravascular catheter manipulation: feasibility of both active and passive tracking in experimental study and initial clinical applications. Radiat Med 2002; 20(1):1–8.

21. Koji I, Daisuke Y, Hironobu I, et al. Hydrodynamic active catheter with multi degrees of freedom motion. IFMBE Proceedings. In World Congress on Medical Physics and Biomedical Engineering, 2006, vol. 14. (Springer Berlin Heidelberg, 2007). p. 3091–4.

Index

Note: Page numbers of article titles are in **boldface** type.

Cardiol Clin 27 (2009) 549–553
doi:10.1016/S0733-8651(09)00048-4
0733-8651/09/$ – see front matter © 2009 Elsevier Inc. All rights reserved.

Printed and bound by CPI Group (UK) Ltd, Croydon, CR0 4YY

03/10/2024

01040362-0017